DIETING
SUCKS
FOR
WOMEN OVER
40

30 TO LIFE

THE ULTIMATE WEIGHT LOSS AND HORMONE BALANCING SOLUTION

Author Info
Email: Debbie@30toLife.org

Publisher Info
Email: support@actiontakerspublishing.com
Website: www.actiontakerspublishing.com

ISBN # (paperback) 978-1-956665-81-9
ISBN # (Kindle) 978-1-956665-82-6
Published by Action Takers Publishing™

READER BONUS!

Dear Reader,

As a thank you for your support, I would like to offer you a special reader bonus. If you've ever been on a diet and haven't been able to sustain it, this download is perfect for you.

Go to https://30toLife.org or click the QR code below and download the 30-Day Balanced Warrior Journal today.

Throughout this book, I will refer to the 30-Day Balanced Warrior Journal. Note that this is NOT a diet regimen. This is a lifestyle change. If you follow this book and commit to becoming healthy, you will. The journal is one of the many tools available to you. My commitment to you: Follow the steps, use the Resources, and you WILL reach your ideal weight and stay there.

Are you ready to live the life you truly want to live? Are you ready to leave that fat behind once and for all and step into your warrior phase of life? Let's do it together.

READER BONUS!

This book is dedicated to my eight-year-old self. You didn't know then how strong you really were. This is for the little girl who just wanted to feel good in her body, be seen, and be loved exactly as she was. You didn't need fixing. You needed kindness, safety, and someone to say, "You matter." I see you now. I've got you.
You Were a Warrior — Your Journey Was Real!

Acknowledgements

This book would not exist without the incredible people who walked alongside me on this journey, cheering, guiding, nudging, and sometimes just quietly holding space while I figured it out.

To Lynda Sunshine West and Action Takers Publishing, thank you for believing in this message and helping me bring it to life with purpose, professionalism, and heart.

To David Mayne, my husband and my rock, thank you for being the tech genius, the event planner, the grounding force, excellent cook, and the one who reminds me daily what balance really means. Your love and support are woven into every page of this book.

To Michael Beas and Atlas Elite Publishing, thank you for showing me what else it takes to launch a book into the world and helping me stretch into what's possible.

To every phenomenal woman who has crossed my path over the past two years — clients, colleagues, friends, and fellow warriors. This book is for you. Your stories, strength, and resilience shaped every chapter.

ACKNOWLEDGEMENTS

A special thank you to Natalie Farnan Gould, your own publishing adventures lit the way for mine. Your enthusiasm, insight, and generous spirit have been a constant source of inspiration.

From the bottom of my heart, thank you.

TABLE OF CONTENTS

Introduction

Dieting sucks. It's time we said it out loud. If you came to this book looking for a magic bullet to lose all your weight, you might just find it here, though it's not magic. It's a life-changing approach that helps you break free from the diet-go-round and finally live without guilt or shame around food. Imagine enjoying eating again... without the emotional baggage.

STOP!

I know, you're already eyeballing the 30-Day Balanced Warrior phase. You're ready to grab your keys, snap a picture of the food list, and run to the grocery store. You're ready to get the show on the road and release your excess weight once and for all. That is exactly what I would do—and did—dozens of times with dozens of books.

Take a breath.

I want you to be successful at reaching your Ideal Healthy Weight (IHW), feeling fantastic, looking younger, and, most importantly, staying there while finding peace with food.

To make that happen, read this book from beginning to end. Take notes. Highlight what hits home. Check out the tools and videos on my Resource Center at https://30toLife.org. And when you're ready…

Let's change your life.

The Three Phases of Your Journey

Phase One – Balanced Warrior

Your 30-Day Balancing phase. Here, we start to calm the chaos, especially around hormones, with a focus on cortisol.

Cortisol is a hormone your body releases in response to stress. It helps regulate blood sugar, metabolism, inflammation, and even your sleep-wake cycle. But when cortisol stays high too long, thanks to chronic stress, it can lead to belly fat, cravings, fatigue, and hormone imbalance.

Check the Resource Center often, watch the videos, and use your Balanced Warrior Journal however it best supports you.

Phase Two – Harmony Heroine

Whew, you made it through Phase I! Now, as a Harmony Heroine, you'll start reintroducing healthy foods while paying attention to how your body responds. You'll continue releasing weight if you haven't hit your IHW yet.

Keep journaling, check the Resource Center, and let this phase feel empowering.

Phase Three – Freedom Eater

WOOHOO!!! Welcome home.

This phase isn't a destination; it's your new lifestyle. As a Freedom Eater, you'll live in a rhythm of balance, ease, and flexibility. You'll learn the 80/20 lifestyle that's allowed me to maintain my IHW long term without the stress, the shame, or the restriction.

Who this book is for.

This book is written with women 40 and older in mind. The societal, emotional, and physical challenges tied to weight are different for women, especially in this stage of life. If you have struggled with your weight all your life, at certain times in your life, or you woke up one morning and suddenly didn't recognize your body, you are in the right place. In order to allow your body to release weight, reduce aches and pains, minimize menopause symptoms, help you get a great night's sleep, and all around feel GREAT, we will start by balancing stress hormones, particularly cortisol! REMINDER: By reading through this entire book, you will know how to reach your ideal healthy weight and stay there easily and effortlessly. No more wasting time, money, and energy on the next best diet. You are already an expert at that, right?

That said, the steps outlined here work for anyone, male or female, at any age. There's even a chapter specifically for men, as women often inspire their partners to make lifestyle changes. The advice is the same, but the approach can differ.

My passion lies with women like me: those who have struggled with their weight for years, yo-yo dieted, and hit a wall when menopause arrived.

Hormone balancing isn't a new concept, but it's been overlooked in mainstream weight-loss conversations for years. Women over 40 know the frustration of doing "everything right" and still not seeing results. That's because traditional diets ignore hormones' critical role in weight management.

Your body isn't just a calorie-burning machine; it's a complex network of systems regulated by hormones like cortisol, insulin, leptin, and ghrelin. These hormones influence everything from how your body stores fat to how hungry you feel. When they're out of balance, often due to stress, poor sleep, or the wrong food choices, releasing weight becomes an uphill battle.

This book doesn't just address what you eat; it addresses how your body responds to it. By focusing on hormone balancing in the first 30 days, we set the stage for long-term, sustainable weight release. And if you're taking prescription medications like GLP-1 receptor agonists (e.g., Ozempic or Wegovy), balancing your hormones becomes even more essential. These drugs can help with appetite control, but they don't fix the underlying imbalances that often lead to weight regain once you stop taking them. I will help you reframe your mindset and deal with your head, not just your body.

Balancing your hormones is the foundation of this program, giving you the tools to work with your body, not against it, for a healthier, slimmer, and more balanced life.

This book will show you how to maintain your weight release, enhance the results of any prescription drugs or surgical treatments, and improve your overall relationship with food and your body. While these drugs can be helpful under the guidance of a medical professional, most people benefit more from understanding their bodies, eating a healthy diet, taking the right supplements, and incorporating movement. The choice to use such medications is personal, and this book is here to support you no matter your path.

What This Book Covers

- In Part 1, we look at where you are now … without judgment.

- In Part 2, we reframe the idea of weight loss to shift your mindset to a healthy lifestyle that is hormonally balanced and allows you to stay at your ideal healthy weight easily and effortlessly.

- Part 3 answers common questions on specific food topics.

- In Part 4, we look at a few of the common challenges people face, especially in the 30-day period, but at other times, too.

- Part 5 is the 30-day Balanced Warrior plan. We begin with a 30-day reset, then move to reintroducing foods, and finally end with an 80/20 lifestyle eating plan.

- Part 6 provides a series of critical support tools that will help you understand and reframe your relationship with food.

- Because most of the book focuses on women, in Part 7, I address a few topics specific to men and children and summarize the book.

- Part 8 has recipes for the Balanced Warrior 30-Day Balancing period and when to add foods back in. Once your body is balanced, these recipes will add to your new healthy eating.

At the end of each short chapter, there is space to take notes and reflect on Your Journey.

What you will experience/how you will benefit

If you are sick and tired of trying new diets, joining another gym, and fed up with feeling frustrated, depressed, and fat, this book will end that cycle forever. Whether you have dieted all your life or woke up one morning wondering where your waistline went, this book will give you the answers to a new, healthy lifestyle. You will live your life diet-free. You will understand how to eat the foods you want to eat. You will have the incredibly powerful tool of self-hypnosis at your fingertips. Here is what I love hearing the most, as one of my clients said: "I got my sexy back."

It saddens me when a woman calls and tells me that she had a lap band or some other surgical procedure, and now she has gained back her weight. These women are truly desperate, and as one such client remarked, "They didn't teach me anything."

I have colleagues who preach that no amount of ice cream, chocolate, French fries, or pizza should ever be consumed. Not ever. But I disagree. Food is more than just fuel for our bodies. It is love, connection, tradition, memory, and celebration. This book isn't about DIE-ting; it is about living with healthy food choices.

> *ProTip*: Your story is your power. Reflect on your relationship with food and the moments that shaped it, not to dwell on the past, but to understand how you've arrived at this chapter of your life. You can't change the beginning, but you have the power to rewrite the rest.

Disclaimer

The information in this book, Dieting Sucks for Women Over 40, is intended for educational and informational purposes only. It is not a substitute for professional medical advice, diagnosis, or treatment.

While I share personal experiences, client stories, and strategies that have worked for me and others, everybody is different. Before making any changes to your diet, exercise routine, medication, supplements, or lifestyle, especially if you have a medical condition, are pregnant, or are taking prescription medications, please consult your physician or qualified healthcare provider.

The author and the publisher do not promise or guarantee weight loss or health outcomes in this book. Your journey is your own, and success depends on many individual factors, including your commitment, consistency, and support system.

I'm not a doctor, nutritionist, or therapist. I'm a coach, a guide, and someone who's walked the walk. I'm here to encourage you, not prescribe anything.

You are responsible for your own health and well-being. You've got this, and when in doubt, ask for help from the professionals you trust.

My Journey

What brought you to this book? Reflect on your personal struggles and goals with weight loss. What are you hoping to gain from this journey?

_____

_____

_____

_____

_____

_____

_____

_____

_____

_____

_____

_____

_____

_____

_____

PART 1

START WHERE
YOU ARE

1

CHAPTER 1

Your Weight Loss Journey

---

*"It's never too late to be what you might
have been."* — George Eliot

Every journey begins somewhere. In Chapter 4, I will share my ups and downs, as well as my own struggles with food, weight, and finding balance. Right now, it's time to turn the lens inward and focus on your journey.

Think back to all the weight loss programs, books, exercise routines, and supplements you've tried. What was happening in your life at the time? For example, I did Weight Watchers, but didn't stop there. I also did Atkins, Keto, HCG Shots, Fat Loss Diet, 20/30 Fast Track, and the list goes on. This isn't an exercise in regret. It's about recognizing your patterns, how your emotions, life circumstances, and relationship with food are all connected.

What has your relationship with food been like? Have you had moments of success, setbacks, frustration, or triumph? This is your opportunity to explore where you've been so you can better understand how to move forward.

Take 10 to 15 minutes to complete this section, then look it over closely to see if you notice any patterns.

Weight loss attempts/diet list	What was happening in my life?
Example: The Diet Center	Example: Before my first wedding
Example: HCG shots	Example: Beginning menopause

We will have some fun with this in Chapter 3:

What is your relationship with food?

- How many diets have you been on?

- How many times have you lost weight, only to gain it back?

- What foods bring you joy? (You know the question: What would you choose for your last meal? For me, it's probably an endless supply of sushi rolls.)

More importantly, can you pinpoint when your relationship with food began to influence your life in meaningful ways? Was it during childhood, adolescence, or adulthood?

For many of us, food is deeply tied to emotions, memories, and traditions. The challenge is that, somewhere along the way, those ties can become complicated. Food shifts from being a source of nourishment to a source of comfort, stress, or even control.

We all have a relationship with food; it's unavoidable. Unlike other habits, food isn't something you can quit cold turkey. Even fasting, though temporarily effective, doesn't teach us anything except how to feel hungry. Have you ever paused to reflect on where your relationship with food began? Was it when someone told you to "clean your plate because children are starving somewhere"? Or perhaps when dessert became a reward for finishing vegetables? Or when family members pushed second helpings onto you to avoid offending them? For many of us, food became tied to guilt, obligation, and even punishment.

At the same time, food is love. It's tied to happy memories: a favorite dish from a beloved relative, the smell of a holiday meal, or baking cookies with kids. Take a moment to reflect on your earliest food memories, both the joyful and the difficult ones. You may find some associations that aren't happy, and that's okay. Be kind to your younger self. That child was doing their best with the tools they had.

A Relaxation Exercise to Help Explore

To truly reflect on your journey, it's helpful to be in a relaxed, open state of mind. Here's a simple relaxation technique you can use anytime to calm your thoughts and explore these memories with clarity:

1. Sit comfortably with your feet flat on the floor.
2. Take a few deep breaths using the 4-7-8 breathing technique:

    -   Breathe in through your nose for 4 seconds.
    -   Hold your breath for 7 seconds.
    -   Slowly exhale through your mouth for 8 seconds.
    -   Repeat 4 times.

As you feel your body and mind begin to relax, gently let your thoughts drift back to your earliest food memories. When did food start to take on an emotional role in your life?

If you want to get into a deeper, relaxed state, go to my website for some free meditation: https://30toLife.org.

Here are some common themes I've heard from clients:

-   "You can't have dessert unless you finish everything on your plate."
-   "Grandma will be upset if you don't take seconds."
-   "There are starving children in (you fill in the blank)."
-   "You're too thin! You need to eat."
-   Someone called you fat, chubby, or thunder thighs, and it stuck with you.

Take note of any memories that surface. Where do you feel them in your body? Does tension show up in your shoulders, chest, or stomach?

Letting Go of the Past

Now, take a deep breath and remind yourself: it's all okay.

The people who shaped your early experiences with food, whether parents, grandparents, teachers, or peers, were likely doing their best with what they knew at the time. Their intentions may have been kind, even if their words or actions left lasting impressions.

But here's the good news: you are in control now.

You have the power to redefine your relationship with food. By reflecting on your past without judgment, you're taking the first step toward freeing yourself from habits and beliefs that no longer serve you.

If this reflection stirs up difficult emotions, that's okay too. Sometimes our relationship with food is tied to deeper emotional experiences. If you feel overwhelmed, I encourage you to reach out to a counselor, therapist, or trusted professional who can help you work through these feelings in a safe and supportive way.

Moving Forward

Now that you've explored your journey, take a moment to honor where you've been. Every success, every setback, and every lesson has brought you to this moment.

In the next chapter, we'll focus on where you're going. What drives you to make this change? What's your Why? Let's uncover it together.

> *ProTip*: Your story is your power. Reflect on your relationship with food and the moments that shaped it. Do not to dwell on the past, but understand how you've arrived at this chapter of your life. You can't change the beginning, but you have the power to rewrite the rest.

Reflection is a tool, not a punishment. Use it to understand the 'why' behind your habits without judgment. Try keeping a food and mood journal for a week, write down what you eat and how you feel before and after meals. You might uncover patterns that offer surprising insights into your relationship with food. Remember, awareness is the first step to change. I know that keeping a food journal may remind you of past "diets" that suggested the same thing. Look at this 30-Day Balanced Warrior Journal as pure fun and exploration.

You Are a Warrior — Your Journey Is Real!

Download your 30-Day Balanced Warrior Journal by going to https://30toLife.org.

My Journey

Where have you been on your own weight release journey? Reflect on moments of success, setbacks, and how your relationship with food has evolved over time.

_____

_____

_____

_____

_____

_____

_____

_____

_____

_____

_____

_____

_____

_____

CHAPTER 2

Emotional Triggers

"It takes a great deal of bravery to stand up to our enemies, but just as much to stand up to our friends."
— JK Rowling, *Dumbledore, Harry Potter and the Sorcerer's Stone*

Triggers are events, situations, smells, tastes, words, or activities that elicit a reaction before we even realize we're reacting. My seven-year-old self, for example, would slam the bathroom door and cry for hours when my father didn't show up again.

In that moment, the trigger was disappointment: a sudden change in plans, a feeling of abandonment. Years later, I found myself feeling emotional, clingy, and needy every time my husband traveled for work. That familiar feeling of being "left" was overwhelming, even though my reaction had nothing to do with the present situation.

Have you ever had someone ask a question, make a comment, or even look at you a certain way, and suddenly, you're reacting in a way that feels disproportionate to the situation? Those are your triggers, or, as they're often called, your "buttons."

Recognizing Your Triggers

Think about your own triggers. When was the last time you reacted strongly to something, only to later wonder, "Why did I react that way?" Often, our closest relationships set the stage for these reactions. It makes sense, our early experiences shape the patterns we carry into adulthood. Without consciously recognizing and addressing these patterns, we will likely repeat them.

Let's be clear: this book isn't about psychoanalysis or therapy. We're not diving deep into the past to unearth every root cause. But recognizing your triggers can provide powerful insights into the buttons that get pushed. Once you acknowledge them, you can start negotiating with your younger self, reminding her that these triggers no longer serve you in the present.

Your Subconscious: A Four-Year-Old at the Wheel

As a certified hypnotist, I've learned that our subconscious mind always works to serve our best interests. The challenge is that our subconscious operates at the emotional level of a four-year-old. A four-year-old wants to be loved, feel safe, secure and accepted. As we mature, those desires do not change; however, the way we reach for them may.

Take cigarette smoking, for example. Think back to a schoolyard scene: a circle of kids smoking together. For the subconscious, i.e., a four-year-old, this represents inclusion, acceptance, and belonging. As teenagers, we associate all these positive emotions with being "cool." Being included in the "in" or "popular" clique. Emotionally speaking, the four-year-old and the teenager are similar. Intellectually speaking, the teenager probably knows that smoking doesn't make you cool. You are cool without smoking. When we allow our subconscious to control our conscious, oftentimes there's hell to pay (or food to eat).

Now fast-forward 20 years. You know smoking isn't cool; it's harmful to your health. But your subconscious doesn't make that distinction. Its primary goal is to keep you happy, and it remembers that smoking once made you feel included and accepted.

The same is true for food. If eating calmed you, made you feel safe, or helped you feel connected as a child, your subconscious will continue to reach for food whenever you're stressed, lonely, or nervous. Unlike cigarettes, though, we can't quit food cold turkey. Food is with us from the very beginning of life, it's fundamental.

"Eat to live; don't live to eat." — Socrates

Your subconscious doesn't care about calories, weight, or health. It just wants to keep you happy. And when food is tied to feelings of comfort and safety, dieting feels like negotiating with a determined four-year-old.

Why Diets Feel Impossible

Dieting isn't about willpower or discipline but understanding your subconscious. I repeat: Dieting isn't about willpower or discipline; it's about understanding your subconscious. You're not failing at dieting; you're simply up against a part of yourself that's working overtime to protect you.

One strategy to manage this inner four-year-old is distraction. When a child is upset, we often redirect their attention. In the same way, we can redirect our subconscious toward healthier habits and patterns.

Start by removing the negative self-talk. The key is to catch yourself when thoughts like "I'm a failure" or "I can't do this" creep in. Replace them with neutral or positive phrases. A trick I learned from a dear friend is to say "Cancel" whenever a negative thought sneaks in. It's a small step, but it helps shift your mindset over time.

Words Matter: Release, Don't Lose

Consider what happens when you lose something, like your keys or phone. You frantically search for it, growing more frustrated with each passing minute. Now, imagine your subconscious behaving the same way when you "lose" weight. That's why I encourage you to re-place the word "lose" with "release." When you release weight, your subconscious won't try to "find" it again.

This shift in language may seem small, but it can have a profound impact. Words shape how we think and feel, and this subtle change tells your subconscious that you're letting go of something you no longer need, not misplacing something you want back.

Kindness Is Key

Releasing weight, changing eating habits, and breaking lifelong pat-terns isn't easy. But it's not about perfection or ease, it's about prog-ress. Be kind to yourself. Imagine speaking to your younger self: what would you say to comfort and encourage her?

Now, offer that same kindness to your current self.

Food is life. It's meant to be joyous, fun, and nourishing. This journey isn't about deprivation; it's about learning to enjoy food while aligning it with your goals.

Keep reading. You are discovering how to reach your ideal healthy weight naturally and stay there easily and effortlessly.

You Are a Warrior — Your Journey Is Real!

ProTip: Emotional triggers are opportunities for growth, not setbacks. When a trigger arises, pause and acknowledge it rather than reacting impulsively. A deep breath or a quick mental reset can help you regain control. This takes practice. I still respond to certain "buttons," but beat myself up less. Self-kindness is Key. Replace phrases like "I can't do this" with empowering alternatives such as "I am learning and growing daily." Use visualization to picture yourself handling triggers with grace and strength. Remember, shifting how you respond to triggers is a decisive step in transforming your relationship with food and yourself.

You Are a Warrior — Your Journey Is Real!

My Journey

What emotions tend to drive your eating patterns? Reflect on the last time you ate due to stress, sadness, or even happiness, and how you might respond differently.

_____

_____

_____

_____

_____

_____

_____

_____

_____

_____

_____

_____

_____

_____

CHAPTER 3

Match Your List

"I realize it has become too easy to find a diet to fit in with whatever you happen to feel like eating and that diets are not there to be picked and mixed but picked and stuck to, which is exactly what I shall begin to do once I've eaten this chocolate croissant." —Helen Fielding, *Bridget Jones's Diary*

How many different diets have you tried? Let's have some fun with this. Again, no judgment. Please take a moment to think about it. Here's my list, and I may have forgotten a few from the 50+ years I spent riding the diet train. Some of these I tried multiple times. I was always ready for the next big thing, convinced that this one would be the answer.

Looking back at this list, I see hundreds, probably thousands, of dollars spent, countless hours of effort, fleeting moments of success, far too many failed attempts, and years of frustration.

My Diet List:

- Weight Watchers
- Master Cleanse
- Isagenix
- Herbalife
- Jenny Craig
- Nutrisystem
- Weigh In
- The Diet Center
- Beverly Hills Diet
- Fit for Life
- Zone Diet
- Atkins
- Keto
- HCG Shots
- Fat Loss Diet
- 20/30 Fast Track
- Paleo Diet
- Vegan Eating for Weight Loss
- Eat Right for Your Blood Type
- doTERRA Slim & Sassy
- Sunrider
- South Beach Diet

- Subway Diet
- Juice Fasting
- Arbonne Diet
- Gluten-Free Diet
- Candida Diet
- Intermittent Fasting
- Dark Chocolate/Red Wine Diet (I know, this sounds like the best diet ever.)
- 1 Day Off Diet
- Dry Body Brushing for Weight Loss

Your list may look like mine, shorter or longer. Think about how much energy you've put into "trying the next new thing." It's exhausting. The promises, the hopes, the effort, and the inevitable cycle of frustration.

But here's what I want you to do right now:

Congratulate yourself. Really –

You Are a Warrior — Your Journey Is Real!

ProTip: Your list is proof of your dedication to finding what works for you. Instead of chasing the next trend, focus on creating sustainable habits that align with your life and goals. Each diet on your list taught you something, channel those lessons into your long-term strategy. Remember, it's about progress, not perfection. Celebrate the fact that you're investing in yourself.

You Are a Warrior — Your Journey Is Real!

My Journey

Reflect on all the diets you've tried, what worked, what didn't, and how they made you feel. What patterns or lessons can you take from those experiences to guide your next steps? Write down one or two things you'll prioritize moving forward.

_____

_____

_____

_____

_____

_____

_____

_____

_____

_____

_____

_____

_____

CHAPTER 4

Where It All Started

"Fall in love with taking care of yourself."
— Anonymous

My story may or may not resonate with you. I suspect parts of this book will touch a place deep within you. We are all shaped by the times we grew up, the people around us, and the lessons we absorbed. I hope that you'll find clarity here and, most importantly, a path to free yourself from the obsession with food and dieting.

Come along with me on my dieting escapades. I promise some of my stories will make you smile or laugh. As you read, take a moment to reflect on your own experiences. We looked at some of this in Part I. Understanding why and how your relationship with food evolved will help you reach your IHW and stay there easily and effortlessly. Please take a moment to think about these questions. How often were you "on a diet"? When you were "off," what foods did you turn to? How did you feel when you were "good" or "bad," based on whether you followed the rules?

But let's remember there is no judgment. Food is neither good nor bad, and your worth has nothing to do with your weight, past, present, or future. Instead, let's marvel at the ingenuity we've all shown in our quest to release weight…and how we somehow always managed to find it again.

Remember all the weight release programs, books, exercise routines, and supplements you've tried. What was happening in your life at the time? This isn't an exercise in regret. It's about recognizing your patterns, how your emotions, life circumstances, and relationship with food are all connected.

The Diet Go-Round

I know firsthand how exhausting the pursuit of weight release can be, the time, money, and energy spent on diet programs that promise the world but deliver little. My journey began around age 10 or 11. I remember crying to my mom, telling her how much I hated my stomach. I was the "fat kid" in grammar school, carrying a round belly and later enduring the nickname "thunder thighs." Those words stuck with me for decades.

For me, comfort food came in the form of Kraft American cheese slices and plain white bread, stolen from my grandmother's fridge. Looking back, I wasn't craving the flavor, I was seeking comfort. Today, I wish I could reassure that 11-year-old girl that everything would be okay.

Reflection is an act of grace. It allows us to honor our past without judgment. My personal struggles with food and weight likely began with early childhood trauma. At just 18 months old, I underwent heart surgery, followed by a month-long hospital stay. After the surgery, my mother told me to "never mention it to anyone except a doctor." As a child, I didn't understand the secrecy, but the shame left a lasting mark. I still don't get the secrecy as there were no lasting effects. We cannot control the decisions of others.

By elementary school, I was the tallest and heaviest kid in class. My father had left when I was five, moving across the country to chase his dreams in California, leaving behind broken promises and painful memories. Food became my solace. After all, my imperfections were surely why my father left, right?

Like many of us, I carried these emotional scars into adulthood. As a teenager, my mother and I bonded over unhealthy habits, like binge-watching movies while eating frozen Snickers bars. As I reflect on that time, I realize how much pain we both masked with food.

Why am I sharing this with you? Because we all have our stories. Maybe your struggles began in childhood, or perhaps they started later in life, after a pregnancy, during menopause, or after a particularly stressful event. Whatever your story, you're not alone, and it's not too late to change the narrative.

It doesn't matter how you arrived at this moment or picked up this book. What matters is that you're here, ready to explore a new path toward health and balance. Together, we'll uncover the power of your subconscious, the joy of movement, and the freedom of understanding your relationship with food. This journey isn't about deprivation, it's about empowerment.

Let's get started.

You Are a Warrior — Your Journey Is Real!

My first "official" diet began at age 12 when my mom joined Weight Watchers, and I ate what she ate. I still remember the skinny, boiled hot dogs and vegetables that comprised most of our meals. Mustard was allowed, so I slathered it on hot dogs, hard-boiled eggs, chicken, and even vegetables. To this day, I still occasionally reach for spicy brown mustard.

That summer, I released all my excess weight, and for the first time, I felt noticed. I'll never forget the moment when some guys whistled at me from their car, shouting, "Hey, legs!" At sleepaway camp, I wore a bikini, joined activities, and even had my first kiss in a treehouse, a place I never would have climbed before releasing weight. I was happy, confident, and living the dream.

Then summer ended. I visited my dad in California, and within three weeks, I gained all 30 pounds back. My father, who was also overweight, filled our days with Italian food, ice cream, and every treat imaginable at Disneyland and other amusement parks. Maybe it was guilt, or food was his way of showing love. Either way, I went from happy and confident to miserable and ashamed in just one month.

Have you ever experienced something like that? How did it make you feel? Those moments are not about blame or guilt, they're about understanding where we've been and why. If I could whisper something to that 13-year-old girl, it would be: "You are amazing, and you can create any life you want. Don't let this define you." What would you tell your younger self?

The Endless Cycle

Throughout high school, the weight stayed on. Heartbreaks led to comfort food, and comfort food led to more weight. My best friend and I would drive around the neighborhood stalking our ex-boy-friends' houses, only to end the night drowning our sorrows in plates of chicken parmesan.

At age 19, my friend and I decided to take control. We joined a program called Weigh-In (like Weight Watchers) and followed their structured diet of proteins, bread, fruit, and veggies. I remember us walking to Brooklyn College, eating poached eggs at the campus coffee shop, and walking home, a solid two-mile trek each way. Over a few months, we both released over 40 pounds and felt incredible.

But diets rarely address the emotional reasons behind weight gain. The weight crept back within a couple of years, and the rollercoaster began in earnest. I tried everything from Jenny Craig to Atkins, shakes to cleanses, and every new program that promised the answer. Releasing weight wasn't the hard part; keeping it off was.

The Relationship Connection

I've noticed a pattern throughout my life: when I was single, I was thinner. When I was in a relationship, the weight came back. Dating in my 20s meant dinners out, frozen piña coladas, and little thought about healthy eating. Lean Cuisines became my go-to because they were quick, cheap, and easy. In hindsight, they weren't exactly nutritious, but they helped me feel "in control."

Does this resonate with you? Is there a connection between your weight and your relationships? For me, the weight gain often came when I felt comfortable and secure in a relationship. And when my partner decided it was time to get healthy, I'd join him on the latest fad diet.

One diet I'll never forget was The Beverly Hills Diet, two weeks of eating nothing but fruit. I remember sitting on the couch, devouring half a watermelon, seeds and all. While I did release weight, it wasn't sustainable. Was I going to go out to dinner and order half a watermelon? Of course not.

The Turning Point

At age 28, I gained 75 pounds during my pregnancy. I lost it in six months by living on Lean Cuisine and sheer determination. But my dieting struggles continued for decades. I'd feel miserable on a strict diet, but I'd feel equally miserable when I fell off the wagon and felt out of control.

Here's the thing: Dieting can give us a false sense of control. If I could control what went into my mouth, I felt like I could control every other aspect of my chaotic life. Sound familiar? The problem is that no one can live in constant restriction.

At age 61, I discovered the concept of balancing stress hormones to support weight loss. At that time, I weighed 180 pounds. A program called 20/30 Fast Track helped me start that journey, but as time went on, I felt it was overly restrictive and one-size-fits-all. I had begun researching everything I could about hormones, food, and the mind-body connection. I read a book written in 2015 called The Hormone Reset Diet by Sara Gottfried, M.D. My personal experience and the knowledge I was acquiring inspired me to return to school to become an Integrative Nutrition Health Coach at IIN, with one goal: to create a program that works for real women with real lives.

Now in my mid-60s, I finally have a healthy, reasonable relationship with food. It's not perfect, but it works. I've let go of the obsession with control and embraced the idea that health is about balance, not deprivation.

> *ProTip*: Your journey is unique, and your story holds the power to inspire change. Start by being kind to yourself, treating your past with compassion, and your future with excitement. Remember, reflection isn't about regret but understanding where you've been to map out where you're headed. And

no food is "good" or "bad," only opportunities to learn and grow. Practice removing those labeling words for food. This is a perfect example of where I use the word "Cancel." For instance, if I catch myself saying or thinking, "I'm so stupid for eating that donut," I say, "Cancel" and rephrase it positively, like this, "I will achieve my healthy weight goal."

YOU ARE DOING AMAZING!! Keep on going.

You Are a Warrior — Your Journey Is Real.

My Journey

What lessons have you learned from your past experiences with weight release? Take a moment to reflect on what worked, what didn't, and how those experiences have shaped your journey. Spend 5 minutes writing it down.

_____

_____

_____

_____

_____

_____

_____

_____

_____

_____

_____

_____

_____

_____

PART 2

REFRAMING WEIGHT LOSS/ DIETS

CHAPTER 5

Know Your Why

"He who has a why to live can bear almost any how."
— Friedrich Nietzsche, *Twilight of the Idols*

Now that you've reflected on your journey, it's time to look forward. Knowing your why is the key to staying motivated and focused as you move through this process.

What Is Your Why?

Why do you want to release weight? Why are you committing to this journey? Why is now the right time?

When I ask my clients these questions, the first answers are often surface level:

- "I want to feel more comfortable in my clothes."

- "I have a wedding/anniversary/reunion coming up."

- "My knees hurt."

- "I'm tired all the time."

- "My doctor told me I need to lose weight."

These answers are valid, but they're only the beginning. To create lasting change, you need to dig deeper. What lies beneath these initial answers? What is your real Why, which comes from a place of truth and vulnerability?

Discovering Your Deeper Why

Here are some examples of deeper Whys that clients have shared with me:

- "My son/daughter is having a baby. It's my first grandchild, and I want to be around. I want to play on the floor with them and be able to stand up after. I want to see my grandchildren grow up."

- "My family has a history of chronic diseases, heart disease, diabetes, and more. I don't want to follow that path. I want to do everything I can to remain strong and healthy, for myself and my family."

- "I love to travel. I want to visit new places, walk around Europe, climb steps, and keep up with the group without feeling exhausted. I want to enjoy those experiences fully, not feel limited by my body."

- "I believe I can live to 105, and I want to do everything I can to get there, and be in good health when I do."

- "This weight release is for ME. I've struggled all my life with my weight, and once and for all, I want to be in control. I want to prove to myself that I can do this."

Your Why doesn't have to be monumental to anyone but YOU. What matters is that it resonates deeply, giving you strength and focus even on the toughest days.

Staying Connected to Your Why

Your Why may evolve as you progress through this journey. That's natural. What's important is to stay connected to it.

Here are some ways to keep your Why front and center:

1. Write it down daily in the 30-day Balanced Warrior Journal

   - Start each morning by writing or reflecting on your Why. This small act reinforces your motivation and sets a positive tone for the day.

2. Create a visual reminder

   - Make a vision board, save a photo on your phone, or write your Why on a sticky note and place it where you'll see it often.

3. Incorporate it into self-hypnosis

   - As you practice self-hypnosis, include your Why as part of your suggestions. For example:

     o "I am committed to this journey because I am strong, confident, and healthy for my family and myself."

     o Speak in the present tense with your self-hypnosis. More in Chapter 25.

Final Thoughts

Your Why is your anchor. It will guide you through this journey and help you stay committed when motivation wavers.

Take the time to honor your Why, revisit it often, and let it remind you of the life you're building for yourself.

You Are a Warrior — Your Journey Is Real!

ProTip: Your Why is your compass, guiding you through the tough days and keeping you on track. Please write it down and keep it visible on your fridge, your mirror, and your phone. Revisit it often, especially when motivation dips. Bonus: Create a playlist of songs that remind you of your Why and play it when you need a boost. Or make a list of quotes that you have in Notes on your phone. I am a big quote person. They are always there to give me extra motivation.

You Are a Warrior — Your Journey Is Real!

My Journey

What is your "Why"? What drives you to make a change? Write down the deeper motivations behind your desire for health and weight balance.

_____

_____

_____

_____

_____

_____

_____

_____

_____

_____

_____

_____

_____

_____

CHAPTER 6

Less Is Not More

---

*"The trouble with eating Italian food is that five or six
days later, you're hungry again."* — George Miller

One of the biggest challenges I encounter with my clients is their ingrained belief that less is more. If I eat less, I'll lose more weight, right? Wrong. I was the same way. I used to think that cutting calories to the bone would be the fastest way to drop weight. Back then, I lived on a steady diet of salads and Lean Cuisine (how did I ever eat those things?) and washed it all down with Diet Coke. I also drank a ton of TAB. Do you remember the pink can? It was a breakthrough that we had a diet soda to wash down all our unhealthy, fatty foods. Sound familiar?

It made sense at the time. After all, I was in my 20s and early 30s, and I was constantly moving my body. Living in Manhattan in a 6th-floor walk-up meant no quick trips back for an umbrella or forgotten item; I wasn't climbing those stairs again! Add to that staying out all night dancing, and walking everywhere in Manhattan.

I gained 75 pounds during my pregnancy because I was eating all the time, mostly Italian food, if I remember correctly. After my pregnancy, I thought the key to releasing weight was to just eat less. And I mean less. My meals consisted of Lean Cuisine, barely anything else, and I had a husband, house, infant, dog, puppy, and two cats. Needless to say, I didn't sit down a lot in those days. Sure, the weight came off eventually, but here's the thing: it didn't stay off.

And it didn't teach me anything about sustainable, healthy habits.

The "Eat Less" Trap

Maybe you also practiced the living on lettuce routine when you were younger. But let's be honest, how sustainable was it? How many times did it lead to bingeing or obsessing over food? And how often did you end up regaining the weight you lost?

We're beyond that now. We understand that starving ourselves and putting our bodies into "survival mode" is counterproductive. Severe calorie restriction can mess with your metabolism, lead to nutrient deficiencies, and even cause long-term health issues. It's not just about weight; it's about your overall well-being.

Why Starvation Doesn't Work

Here's what happens when you severely restrict calories: Your body thinks it's in a famine. Historically, early humans had to endure long periods without food, so their bodies adapted by slowing down their metabolism to conserve energy. It was a survival mechanism then, but today, it's what makes extreme dieting so ineffective. When your metabolic rate slows down, you burn fewer calories, even at rest. You're working against your body instead of with it.

Not to mention the psychological toll of starvation-mode dieting. Feeling hungry and deprived all the time isn't just unsustainable, it's downright miserable. You're setting yourself up for failure when you're constantly battling cravings, irritability, and the inevitable binge that comes after restriction.

Health Risks of Extreme Calorie Cutting

Let's talk about the risks. Severe calorie restriction isn't just ineffective; it can harm your body. According to Gundersen Health, extreme calorie cutting can lead to muscle loss, nutrient deficiencies, depression, and even increased risk for conditions like diabetes. https://30to-Life.org/references.

When you starve your body, it begins to break down muscle for energy because it lacks sufficient fuel. And here's the kicker: muscle keeps your metabolism running strong. Losing muscle means your metabolism slows down even more, making it harder to lose weight in the long run.

Then there's the mental aspect. Extreme calorie restriction leads to obsession. You become consumed with thoughts of food, what you're allowed to eat, what you're craving, and how many calories you've had. It's exhausting and completely unnecessary.

What You Should Be Doing Instead

The good news? You don't have to live this way anymore. The Lean Cuisine and Diet Coke days are over!

Be sure to eat. That's right, eat! Give your body what it needs: lean protein, fruits, and tons of non-starchy vegetables. Your body craves nutrients, and it thrives when you fuel it with whole, nutrient-dense foods.

This isn't about deprivation; it's about abundance. Load your plate with colorful veggies, fresh fruit, and satisfying protein. Whether you prefer to graze throughout the day, eat three square meals, or practice intermittent fasting, the key is to nourish your body with healthy, balanced meals.

Reframe Your Mindset

Let's reframe how we think about food and weight release:

- Eating less isn't the answer; eating better is.
- Focus on quality, not just quantity.
- Fuel your body, don't starve it.

Remember, weight release isn't just about calories in versus calories out. It's about creating balance, balancing your hormones, balancing your plate, and balancing your lifestyle. When you give your body the nutrients it needs, it rewards you with energy, better sleep, clearer skin, and weight that naturally falls into place.

You Are a Warrior — Your Journey Is Real!

Pro Tip: Nourishment, not deprivation, is the key to sustainable weight release. Forget the "eat less" mentality and focus on eating better. Remember to crowd out less healthy food choices by filling your plate with colorful, nutrient-dense foods, such as lean proteins, fruits, and non-starchy vegetables. Remember, severe calorie restriction slows your metabolism and leads to burnout. Instead, fuel your body to thrive. Quality over quantity always wins.

You Are a Warrior — Your Journey Is Real!

CHAPTER 7

Intermittent Fasting: The Pause That Empowers

"The universe does not have laws. It has habits. And habits can be broken." — Tom Robbins

---

One of the questions I always get is, "Can I intermittent fast during the first 30 days?" My answer? Not usually.

While intermittent fasting (IF) definitely has benefits, I've found it's best to focus on three meals a day during the Balanced Warrior phase. Your body is recalibrating physically, hormonally, and emotionally. The goal isn't restriction. It's nourishment. If you're already fasting before starting the program, you can continue if it feels good. But if you're dealing with blood sugar issues or emotional eating, I generally suggest waiting.

So… What Is Intermittent Fasting?

At its core, intermittent fasting means eating during a set window of time and fasting the rest of the day. It's not starvation. And yes, you can still have your morning coffee. Just skip the cream and sugar if you're in a fasted state. You can use liquid Stevia, and I love a couple of drops of chocolate and peppermint in my morning coffee.

Fasting is far from new. It's been practiced for thousands of years across cultures and religions. In ancient Greece, Hippocrates, often called the father of modern medicine, recommended fasting for healing. In spiritual traditions, fasting has long been used to clear the mind and purify the body. Think of Ramadan in Islam, Yom Kippur in Judaism, Lent in Christianity, or the fasting rituals in Buddhism and Hinduism. I grew up Jewish (but not religious) and, in Brooklyn, all my friends fasted on Yom Kippur. I never did and didn't really understand the reasoning behind it.

"To keep the body in good health is a duty... otherwise
we shall not be able to keep our mind strong and clear."
— Buddha

In Buddhism, especially within the Theravāda tradition, fasting supports mindfulness and reduces attachment to worldly desires. Monks and nuns typically follow a schedule where all meals are consumed before noon, allowing the afternoon and evening to be focused on meditation, study, and spiritual reflection.

Lay Buddhists often observe fasting on Uposatha days, bimonthly days of heightened spiritual practice. They avoid solid food after noon, practice silence, and dedicate time to ethical living and introspection. The goal is never punishment but rather simplicity and awareness.

Fasting is seen as a way to quiet the mind and deepen the connection between body and spirit.

"When you fast, do not look somber as the hypocrites do... but put oil on your head and wash your face, so that it will not be obvious to others that you are fasting."
—Matthew 6:16–18

In Christianity, fasting is seen as a profoundly spiritual discipline to humble oneself, seek clarity, and draw closer to God. It's mainly observed during Lent, 40 days of reflection and repentance leading to Easter. Many Christians fast on Ash Wednesday and Good Friday, often giving up specific foods or pleasures as a form of sacrifice. The intent isn't punishment, but spiritual focus. Fasting in Christianity is about aligning the heart with divine purpose, quieting distractions, and making space for prayer, reflection, and renewal.

"Afflict your souls on the tenth day of the seventh month."
— Leviticus 16:29 (Yom Kippur fasting)

Fasting in Judaism is rooted in both historical remembrance and personal reflection. While Yom Kippur, the Day of Atonement, is the most well-known fast, several others are observed throughout the Jewish calendar, including Tisha B'Av (mourning the destruction of the Temples), the Fast of Esther, and the Tenth of Tevet. These fasts vary in length but share common intentions: repentance (teshuvah), humility, and reconnection with faith. Prayer, study, and acts of charity often accompany fasting. It is seen as a sacred pause, a way to step back from the physical world and re-center on spiritual values.

"There is no possibility of one's becoming a yogi... if one eats too much, or eats too little, sleeps too much or does not sleep enough." — Bhagavad Gita, Chapter 6, Verse 16

In Hinduism, fasting is a common practice that varies widely across regions, traditions, and deities. It is often observed on specific days of the week, during festivals like Navratri, or in devotion to deities such as Shiva or Vishnu. Some fasts involve complete abstinence from food, while others allow fruits, nuts, and milk. The spiritual purpose of fasting in Hinduism is to purify the body and mind, exercise discipline, and strengthen one's connection to the divine. It is viewed not as deprivation, but as a sacred offering, an intentional pause to refocus energy inward.

In these traditions, fasting isn't about weight release. It's about reflection, discipline, and renewal. So, while intermittent fasting might feel trendy now, its roots run deep.

The Science of the Fast

When we fast, a few things happen inside the body:

- Insulin levels drop, allowing your body to access stored fat more easily.

- Human growth hormone increases, which can support fat burning and muscle maintenance.

- Cellular repair begins, including a process called autophagy, which is your body's way of cleaning out damaged cells.

- Inflammation decreases, which may reduce the risk of chronic disease.

If it's done mindfully, many women over 40 find IF especially helpful for regulating blood sugar, improving energy, and calming hormonal chaos. While this is true, I have worked with clients who are taking insulin, and IF is not recommended in this case, even though balancing your hormones can and does improve blood sugar. One client's doctor reduced her insulin by half during the initial 30 days of the Balanced Warrior phase simply because of what she was eating and not eating. This same client wanted to incorporate IF at the beginning, and that was way too dramatic given her insulin dependency. Be mindful of what works for you.

Fasting can also backfire if you're under chronic stress or not sleeping well. Cortisol can spike when your body thinks it's in survival mode. That's why I often suggest waiting until after the 30-day Balanced Warrior phase. You want to be balanced before you try to stretch your eating window.

So, where does that leave you? With options, particularly as you progress to the Harmony Heroine and Freedom Eater phases. Intermittent fasting is a tool, not a rule. If it works for you, great. If not, you've got plenty of other strategies in this book.

My Experience with IF

When I first heard about intermittent fasting, I'll be honest, I didn't think I would like it. It felt like just another trend. Besides, I was a breakfast girl, peanut butter on toast, vegan cheese on a slice of whole grain, simple but satisfying. Also, let's not forget my history with The Master Cleanse, lemon, water, and cayenne. That was a vivid memory about fasting, and it wasn't fun.

And of course, many of us were raised with the idea that "Breakfast is the most important meal of the day." It is still referred to in some cereal marketing. Growing up on Frosted Flakes, Lucky Charms, and Pop-Tarts was not a healthy start to my day. All part of marketing the idea of convenience, and us kids getting a ton of sugar every morning. Adult obesity, diabetes, ADHD, and many other chronic health concerns may be traced back, at least in part, to early and consistent sugar consumption.

My clients continued to ask me about IF, and I am a big believer in trying something so that I can speak to my experience. I started with a 16:8 schedule, eating between noon and 8 p.m. The first few weeks were rough. I missed my morning routine. I drank more coffee than I probably should have (black with a splash of liquid Stevia, which is IF approved). But eventually, I got into the rhythm.

I must admit that I liked how I felt. I wasn't obsessing over food. I had more energy. My weight stayed stable. It felt like freedom from thinking about food as much as usual. Over time, I found that 16/8 was losing its charm, and I returned to a healthy breakfast. I noticed that, just by chance, I was fasting for 12-14 hours on most mornings. That continues to work for me. If you give yourself a good 12 hours, you are intermittent fasting.

You have to find what works for you. There's no one-size-fits-all here, just options that support your life.

Not a Free Pass

Some of my clients find IF liberating. They love knowing when they'll eat and enjoy fewer decisions. But here's the thing: just because you're eating in a specific window doesn't mean nutrition goes out the window. The Freedom Eater lifestyle you're learning in this book can blend nicely with intermittent fasting. Don't use intermittent fasting as an excuse to load up on junk during your eating window.

Start slowly. Be curious. If it doesn't feel right for your body or your lifestyle, skip it.

> ***ProTip***: Start with a 12:12 or 14:10 window. Water is still key, and switch to decaf if you drink more coffee in your fasting hours. Pay attention to your stress levels and your sleep. And most of all, don't use fasting as another way to punish yourself. If it feels wrong, stop. If it feels good, keep going. Your body knows.

You Are a Warrior — Your Journey Is Real!

CHAPTER 8

Making Peace with Food

"Never underestimate how much assistance, how much satisfaction, how much comfort, how much soul and transcendence there might be in a well-made taco."
— Tom Robbins, *Jitterbug Perfume*

Some foods might not be the healthiest choices. But let's face it, cravings for comfort foods are real. You've probably felt it yourself. Maybe you crave chocolate after a stressful day or reach for salty chips when tired. Have you noticed how cravings shift with the seasons or your emotional state? That's not a coincidence.

In fact, there's science to back this up. Fatty and sugary foods, what we call "comfort foods", trigger a temporary reaction in the brain. They soothe or uplift us for a brief moment, creating a sense of calm or happiness. It's fleeting, of course, but it's real.

A 2024 study by the Monell Center offers fascinating insights into these cravings. Researchers studying gut-brain circuits in mice discovered new clues about why we're drawn to sugar and fat and why cutting them out entirely can feel so impossible. (The study is on our Resources page at https://30toLife.org/references.)

So yes, cravings are real. But food is about more than just biology; it's deeply tied to our emotions, memories, and culture.

Food as Love; Food as Memory

Food is love. You've probably heard Chef Emeril Lagasse say it, and I wholeheartedly agree. Food has a way of transporting us to cherished moments. It can evoke powerful memories with a single smell or taste.

Think about it: Is there a food that instantly brings you back to a happy memory? Maybe the smell of freshly baked cookies reminds you of baking with your mom or grandmother. Perhaps it's the taste of a dish your dad made on weekends. Or maybe it's a meal you had during a memorable vacation or family holiday.

One of my clients, a gentleman in his 50s, struggled with a craving for ice cream. Every day when he passed a particular ice cream shop on his way home from work, he found himself in the drive-thru, ordering a cone. When we explored this craving, he realized it stemmed from childhood memories of getting ice cream with his grandfather. That simple cone wasn't about sugar, it was about love, connection, and joy.

Once he understood the memory behind the craving, he didn't have to give up ice cream entirely. Instead, he enjoyed it intentionally, just once a week instead of every day. With that shift, and a few other changes, he began releasing the 30 pounds he wanted to release.

Food, Culture, and Tradition

Food isn't just about personal memories; it's also about culture and tradition. Consider how certain foods are woven into the fabric of celebrations and holidays.

Does pumpkin pie remind you of Thanksgiving? Does fruitcake (love it or hate it!) remind you of Christmas? For me, it's pecan pie, a must-have for Thanksgiving and Christmas.

Maybe your family makes tamales for Christmas Eve, latkes for Hanukkah, or a special lamb dish for Easter. Perhaps you celebrate Rosh Hashanah with honey cake, or the Fourth of July with barbecue and s'mores. Food helps us connect with our families, communities, and cultures.

Even if you didn't grow up with food traditions, you might have created some of your own as an adult. What are the foods that feel special to you?

Balance, Not Deprivation

Here's the thing: I will not tell you that you can never have the foods you crave.

The foods you grew up on, those tied to happy memories, the foods that are part of your culture, all have a place in your life. This is where the 80/20 Freedom Eater lifestyle comes into play. The 80/20 Freedom Eater lifestyle means that 80% of the time, you focus on eating clean, nourishing, hormone-balancing foods, and the other 20% is reserved for flexibility, enjoyment, and occasional indulgences. I go into detail about the 80/20 Freedom Eater lifestyle in Chapter 24. It's a realistic, sustainable way of eating that honors your health goals and your love for food.

These foods can be part of your occasional 20%. Life is meant to be enjoyed, and food is a big part of that.

But let's be mindful. If some of your favorite treats are also emotional trigger foods (foods you can't stop eating once you start), you'll want to approach them with extra caution. That doesn't mean you can't ever have them again.

"Mindfulness is a way of befriending ourselves and our experience." — Tara Brach

---

Tips for Staying Balanced

Here are some practical tips for enjoying special foods while staying in control:

1. **Be Intentional**

   - If it's a holiday or celebration, enjoy a single serving of your favorite dish.

   - Savor every bite. Make it about the experience, not just the food.

2. **Set Boundaries**

   - If you're hosting, send leftovers home with your guests or throw them out. Yes, throw them out. If the food isn't there, it can't tempt you tomorrow.

   - If you're at someone else's house, politely decline leftovers.

3. **Use Self-Hypnosis**

   - Reinforce that you are in control, not the food.

- Practice visualizing yourself enjoying these special treats without guilt or overindulgence.

For self-hypnosis videos, visit the RESOURCES page here https://30toLife.org.

Food and Celebration

Yes, you can enjoy Thanksgiving, Christmas, Rosh Hashanah, Easter, Three Kings Day, July 4th, or any other holiday filled with delicious foods. Depriving yourself of the connection between food, family, and friends during celebrations doesn't make sense.

This 30-day Balanced Warrior balancing phase is not about deprivation. It's about learning balance. It's about creating a lifestyle where food is no longer a source of stress or guilt but something to be enjoyed as part of your life.

Close your eyes for a moment and imagine this:

- You've reached your Ideal Healthy Weight.
- You're sitting down to a holiday meal, surrounded by loved ones.
- You're enjoying your favorite traditional foods, savoring every bite.
- And you're doing it without guilt, anxiety, or self-recrimination.

Can you picture that? That's what balance looks like.

That's what food freedom feels like.

Final Thoughts

Food is more than calories and macros. It's memory, culture, celebration, and connection. While some foods may not be the healthiest, they can still have a place in your life as part of your 80/20 Freedom Eater lifestyle.

So go ahead and enjoy that pumpkin pie, that slice of pizza, or that childhood favorite, mindfully and with joy. Life is meant to be savored.

You Are a Warrior — Your Journey Is Real!

ProTip: Food is connection, celebration, and memory; indulging occasionally is okay. Use the 80/20 rule: Enjoy meaningful, traditional, or nostalgic foods as part of your 20%, and let them nourish your soul as much as your body. Mindfulness is key. Savor every bite, set boundaries with portions, and get rid of leftovers. Savor positive associations between your memory and certain foods; life is sweeter that way. Balance is where freedom lives.

You Are a Warrior — Your Journey Is Real!

My Journey

What is one treat that brings me joy and fits nicely into my balanced lifestyle? (Think about something you genuinely enjoy and can savor without guilt.)

How does allowing myself treats help me stay on track long-term? (Explore how flexibility and enjoyment contribute to consistency.)

What foods have I been avoiding that I enjoy and can eat in balance? Have I attempted to release weight by severely cutting calories? If so, how did that make me feel?

_____

_____

_____

_____

_____

_____

_____

_____

_____

_____

_____

CHAPTER 9

Fear of Failure and Fear of Success

"What would you do if you weren't afraid?"
— Sheryl Sandberg

Have you ever felt stuck between wanting to succeed and fearing what success might bring? Or perhaps you've worried that this attempt to release weight will lead to another heartbreaking cycle of gaining it back? Let me reassure you, you're not alone.

For many of us, weight release isn't just about the scale. It's an emotional journey filled with internal battles that go far beyond food choices or exercise routines. Behind every diet we've tried, every pound gained or lost, there are fears lurking beneath the surface. These fears often fall into two categories: fear of failure and fear of success.

Let's start by acknowledging that these fears are completely normal. You're not broken for feeling them. Recognizing them is the first step toward breaking free from their grip. This book isn't just about what's on your plate; it's about what's going on in your mind and soul. You're embarking on a new way of living, learning to live diet-free, which means addressing the emotional hurdles that might be holding you back.

What Is Fear of Failure?

The Fear of Failure is the overwhelming concern that taking action or pursuing a goal will result in a negative outcome, embarrassment, or disappointment. In the context of weight release, this fear might manifest as:

- Doubts about your ability to stick to the Balanced Warrior
- 30-day balancing plan.
- Anxiety about regaining lost weight.
- Feeling defeated before you've even started because of past experiences.

Maybe you're thinking: "I've tried so many diets before and spent so much money. What if I fail again?" Sound familiar? It certainly did for me. Every new program I tried came with hope, but deep down, that nagging voice was always whispering, "What if it doesn't work? What if I can't keep it off?"

But here's the thing: You're not failing. You've been caught in an endless loop of diets that weren't designed to work long-term. They didn't teach you about your body, your hormones, or how to create a healthy relationship with food. You were set up to fail, and now you're stepping off that rollercoaster for good. This is different. This isn't about deprivation or willpower. It's about building a lifestyle that feels good and works for YOU.

Let's reframe failure for a moment. Failure isn't the end; it's part of the journey. Every "stumble" is a chance to learn something new about your body and your habits. With each step, you're building the tools and resilience to maintain your healthy weight for life.

What Is Fear of Success?

On the flip side, the Fear of Success is the anxiety that achieving your weight release goals will bring about unforeseen challenges or changes. You might wonder:

- "What if I can't maintain this weight?"
- "What if people treat me differently now?"
- "What if I lose this new version of myself the way I've lost weight and gained it back before?"

This fear hit me hard every time I reached my goal weight. I thought, "Now what? How do I keep this up? Can I maintain this without living on lettuce and misery?" Fear of success can be subtle, but it's powerful. It can lead to subconscious resistance, sabotaging your progress before you even realize what's happening.

Sometimes, fear of success can show up in our relationships. Maybe you're afraid that losing weight will shift dynamics with a partner, friend, or family member. Maybe you're worried about receiving too much attention or feeling the pressure to "stay perfect" in the eyes of others. These thoughts can create a mental block that makes success feel overwhelming or even unappealing.

You're not afraid of success. You're scared of what might come with it. The pressure. The attention. The unknown. Change takes us out of our comfort zone. Even if that comfort zone has us wanting to release weight, eat healthier, exercise more, whatever it is. Somewhere deep down, we know that successfully reaching our weight release goal will make us proud, and yet... You shed those excess pounds, and along with them, the version of yourself the world had grown used to. And that's OKAY – the outside doesn't actually change WHO you are.

Success doesn't have to feel scary or temporary. You're creating a sustainable lifestyle that allows for flexibility, joy, and ease. Success doesn't mean perfection; it means finding balance.

Breaking the Cycle

So, how do we move past these fears? First, we recognize that they're normal. They're part of the process of creating lasting change. Then, we work on reframing our mindset and building habits that align with the life we want to live.

1. Replace "Failure" with Growth

What if every stumble was simply an opportunity to learn? Instead of thinking, "I failed because I had a donut," reframe it as, "I learned that having a donut didn't ruin my entire day. I can enjoy a treat and still be in control."

This is where your daily weigh-ins and journaling become so important. We will discuss this in Chapter 21. They help you identify patterns without judgment. You're gathering data about how your body responds, what triggers your cravings, and how you can adjust. You are also developing a lifelong habit of weighing yourself without fear. This will serve you well when you get to the Freedom Eater phase.

2. Use Self-Hypnosis to Combat Fear

Your subconscious is incredibly powerful. When fear creeps in, self-hypnosis can help you replace it with calm, confidence, and control. For example, you might use affirmations like:

- "I am in control of my body and my choices."

- "I am proud of the progress I've made, and I trust myself to maintain it."

- "Every day, I am learning how to live my best, healthiest life."

Practice self-hypnosis daily to reinforce these positive beliefs. Over time, these affirmations will become your automatic response to fear. We address self-hypnosis in Chapter 25.

3. Celebrate Every Victory—Big or Small

When fear of success starts to creep in, counter it by celebrating your progress. Take a moment to acknowledge how far you've come, whether it's loose clothes, better sleep, or simply feeling more energized. Success isn't just about the number on the scale; it's about how you feel.

Why Plateaus Are NOT Failure

Let's talk about plateaus. Many women will hit a point when the scale stops moving or even goes up slightly. This is NORMAL. It's your body adjusting, recalibrating, and balancing. It doesn't mean you've failed or that you'll never release more weight. Life changes are almost always two steps forward, one step back. Have you noticed it in your life? While none of us likes it, it's real. I see it all the time with myself and my clients.

Your body has its own rhythm. Some people release weight steadily daily, while others experience fluctuations or "whooshes" of weight release after a few days of no movement. Trust the process. If you're following the program, the results will come.

Remember, this is a lifestyle, not a sprint. Plateaus are part of the journey, often teaching us patience and resilience. When you hit a plateau, focus on the other wins: Are you feeling stronger? Sleeping better? Is your skin glowing? These are signs that your body is thriving.

Shifting from Fear to Freedom

The goal of this program isn't just to release weight; it's to transform your relationship with food, your body, and yourself. You're breaking free from old habits, yo-yo dieting, and obsession with perfection. You're learning to trust yourself.

Fear of failure and fear of success don't have to define your journey. They're just stepping stones on the path to freedom. And let me tell you, freedom feels amazing.

You Are a Warrior — Your Journey Is Real!

ProTip: Fear is just a thought, not a prediction. You have probably encountered the False Evidence Appearing Real as an acronym for Fear. I always strive to remember that. When fear of failure or success creeps in, pause and acknowledge it without judgment. Write down your worries and challenge them with facts. For example, instead of "What if I gain it all back?" try "I'm learning sustainable habits that support long-term success." Celebrate your progress, whether it's a small victory like drinking more water or a significant milestone like fitting into a favorite outfit. Remember, this is a journey, not a sprint. Every step forward counts.

You Are a Warrior — Your Journey Is Real!

My Journey

What fears of failure or success might be holding you back? Write about how those fears have shown up in your journey and list three ways you might release them.

Fears

_____

_____

_____

_____

3 Ways I Might Release the Fears

1. _____

2. _____

3. _____

CHAPTER 10

Non-Scale Victories

"Success is not the key to happiness. Happiness is the key to success. If you love what you are doing, you will be successful." — Albert Schweitzer

---

You're stepping on the scale every day, and most days, it goes down. Even .2 of a pound is cause for celebration. Remember, this isn't a sprint, it's a marathon. Why? Because you're not just releasing weight; you're recalibrating your body, balancing your hormones, releasing toxins, and creating new habits that will serve you for life.

But then there are those days when the scale doesn't move, or worse, it goes up. Here comes the panic, frustration, and doubt. "What did I do wrong?" you ask yourself. The answer, most often, is simple: nothing. You haven't done anything wrong. Your body is just doing its thing, adapting, adjusting, and finding balance. This journey isn't just about numbers on a scale. It's about progress in all forms. And progress shows up in many ways that aren't tied to a number.

Let me introduce you to the magic of Non-Scale Victories (NSVs).

What Are Non-Scale Victories?

Non-scale victories are the moments of progress that can't be measured in pounds or ounces. They're the subtle (and not-so-subtle)

signs that your body is healing, your habits are changing, and your life is improving. These victories are just as important, if not more important, than the number on the scale.

Here are some common NSVs my clients have reported:

- Feeling physically better: "My knees don't hurt when I climb the stairs anymore!"

- Clothes fitting differently: "I can finally zip up that pair of jeans that's been sitting in my closet for years."

- Glowing skin: "My skin is clearer, and I look so much brighter in the mirror."

- Improved sleep: "I'm finally sleeping through the night, no tossing and turning!"

- More energy: "I don't feel like I need a nap at 3 p.m. anymore."

- Reduced pain: "My back pain is gone, and I feel lighter on my feet."

- Stabilized mood: "I'm less irritable, and my mood swings have disappeared."

- Better endurance: "I walked farther and faster than I have in years!"

- Improved health metrics: Blood pressure, blood sugar, cholesterol, and insulin levels are normalizing.

- Freedom from cravings: Sugar and salt cravings fading away.

- Medication reduction: I got rid of my blood pressure or other meds.

The list goes on. These victories may feel small in the moment, but they add up to something massive: evidence that you are becoming the healthiest version of yourself.

Why Non-Scale Victories Matter

The scale is just one tool in your weight-release journey. It's a guide, not a judge, jury, or executioner. It doesn't tell the whole story of what's happening inside your body. Focusing only on the number makes it easy to get discouraged when it doesn't cooperate. NSVs remind you that progress isn't linear and that the scale doesn't define your success.

Here's the truth: Your body is changing, even if the scale doesn't show it daily. You're releasing inflammation, improving digestion, balancing hormones, and building healthier habits.

NSVs are the proof.

How to Track Your NSVs

I encourage you to start paying attention to these victories and, even better, write them down. Keeping a journal of your progress will remind you how far you've come, especially on the tough days when the scale feels like your enemy. Get the Balanced Warrior 30-Day Journal here https://30toLife.org. Here are some tips for tracking your NSVs:

1. Start a "Victory Journal": Jot down at least one non-scale victory each day. It could be as simple as "drank all my water" or "noticed my rings are looser."

2. Celebrate the small stuff: It's not just about the big milestones. Did you walk an extra block today? Did you resist that cookie craving without even thinking about it? Write it down.

3. Take photos: Progress photos can be a powerful visual reminder of how your body is transforming, even if the scale is stubborn.

4. Measure inches: Sometimes, the scale doesn't move because you're building muscle and losing fat simultaneously. Measuring your waist, hips, arms, and thighs can reveal changes the scale can't.

5. Listen to your body: Notice how you feel, lighter, less bloated, stronger, and more energetic. These feelings are just as important as the physical changes.

Your Journey; Your Victories

No two journeys are the same. Your body is unique, and your progress will look different from that of anyone else. That's why NSVs are so important; they keep the focus on you and your personal growth. Comparing yourself to others only takes away from your achievements. Instead, compare yourself to where you were yesterday, last week, or last month. That's where the magic is.

What Happens When You Reach Your Goal?

One of the most exciting things about NSVs is that they don't stop when you reach your ideal healthy weight. In fact, they often multiply. You'll notice that greasy, fried foods don't appeal to you anymore because they make you feel bloated. You'll crave vegetables because they leave you feeling light and energized. You'll choose movement because it feels good, not because you're forcing yourself to burn calories.

You'll also find that the Freedom Eater 80/20 lifestyle becomes second nature. You'll indulge in your 20% without guilt because your 80% keeps you grounded. The weight will stay off easily and effortlessly because you've built a foundation of habits that support your health and happiness.

A Word on Mindset

As you celebrate your NSVs, remember to keep your mindset strong. Continue practicing self-hypnosis, affirmations, or whatever tools resonate with you. Remind yourself daily that this isn't just about weight; it's about creating a life that feels good, inside and out. The scale is just one piece of the puzzle. The rest? That's your vitality, confidence, and ability to live life to the fullest.

Remember: The Lean Cuisine and Diet Coke days are over. You're not chasing quick fixes or numbers on a scale. You're chasing a healthier, happier, more balanced you.

Celebrate your non-scale victories. They are proof that you're transforming not just your body but your entire life. You've got this!

> ***ProTip***: Non-scale victories (NSVs) are potent reminders that progress is more than just numbers. Focus on how your clothes fit, your energy levels, or the freedom from cravings. Track your NSVs in a journal or celebrate them mentally; every victory, big or small, proves you're on the right path. Non-scale victories are great affirmations for your self-hypnosis. Remember, weight release is about transformation, not perfection.

You Are a Warrior — Your Journey Is Real!

My Journey

What are three positive changes I've noticed that have nothing to do with the scale?" (Think about energy levels, mood, sleep, strength, or how your clothes fit.)

How has focusing on non-scale victories changed how I feel about my progress?" (Has it made the journey more enjoyable or less stressful?)

What is one thing I can celebrate about myself today, no matter how small?" (Remember, every step forward is worth recognizing!)

Run, don't walk, to the Balanced Warrior 30-Day Journal and start your new lifestyle journey today: https://30toLife.org.

_____

_____

_____

_____

_____

_____

_____

_____

_____

_____

PART 3

SPECIFIC FOOD ISSUES?

CHAPTER 11

Cocktails?

"Shaken, not stirred." – James Bond, *Goldfinger* (1964)

The Role of Alcohol

One of the first questions I get from clients is about alcohol. My male clients typically ask, "When can I have my bourbon or beer again?" while my female clients tend to ask, "When can I have my wine or vodka tonic?"

It's a valid concern. For many of us, alcohol isn't just about the drink itself; it's tied to rituals, social interactions, and moments of relaxation. Personally, I enjoy wine, the occasional beer, and exploring different martinis. If drinking alcohol isn't your thing, you are ahead of the game.

But during your Balanced Warrior 30-day balancing phase, you will not be having any alcohol whatsoever.

Yes, I know. That sounds daunting. But trust me, this break is crucial for resetting your body and making real progress toward your Ideal Healthy Weight (IHW). Alcohol is essentially liquid sugar and cutting it out during this phase will help your body recalibrate faster.

Why the 30 Days Matter

Let's get straight to it: alcohol has a significant impact on weight release. It's not just the empty calories; it's how alcohol affects your metabolism, hormones, and appetite. Alcohol disrupts your body's fat-burning process and often triggers cravings for carbs or salty snacks. I always find myself wanting to eat more if I am having alcohol. For some, it has the opposite effect, which means you could deprive your body of much-needed healthy protein. Either way, you want to avoid all alcohol for the Balanced Warrior 30-day balancing phase. You may also want to avoid it until you reach your ideal healthy weight – that's what I did.

During the balancing phase, your body is resetting. Cutting out alcohol ensures that you're giving your body the best chance to adjust, release weight, and stabilize your hormones without interference.

For me, it was 6.5 months before I reintroduced alcohol, and even then, I did it slowly and systematically, just like I reintroduced foods.

Tips for Surviving 30 Days Without Alcohol

If you enjoy alcohol, giving it up for even a short time might feel overwhelming. But here are some tips to help you navigate those moments:

1. **Avoid Tempting Situations**: For the 30 days, it's best to avoid situations where alcohol will be a major focus. Happy hours,

dinner parties, or events where everyone's sipping cocktails can be challenging, especially at first.

2. **Create a Tactile Experience**: One of the things we enjoy about drinking isn't just the taste, it's the ritual. The feel of the glass, the social atmosphere, and the act of holding a drink can all be part of the experience.

Here's what I suggest: grab a stemmed glass (yes, I am adamantly opposed to non-stemmed glasses!) and fill it with something fun but non-alcoholic. If non-stemmed glasses don't bother you, get one of those. The key is the tactile sensation. Try sparkling water, seltzer, or Zevia soda, and garnish it with a slice of lemon, lime, or orange.

Holding that glass in your hand, especially in a social setting, can help you feel included while staying on track.

3. **Practice Saying No**: If someone offers you a drink, have a response ready. Something as simple as "I'm taking a break from alcohol for now" works perfectly. It's pretty common to hear this. Most people won't push further; if they do, smile and stick to your plan.

Reintroducing Alcohol After 30 Days

Once you've completed the Balanced Warrior 30-day balancing phase, and especially if you're still working toward your Ideal Healthy Weight, once again, my suggestion is to hold off on alcohol a little longer.

When you're ready to reintroduce it, proceed slowly and systematically. Your tolerance will likely be lower, and your body will react differently now that it's healthier and more balanced. Here's how to do it:

4. **Start with One Type of Alcohol at a Time**:

   - Introduce one type of liquor, wine, beer, or bubbly at a time.

   - Wait 3-4 days before trying something else to see how your body responds.

5. **Be Mindful of Mixers**:

   - Skip the sugary mixers, which can wreak havoc on your progress. Instead, opt for:

     o Club soda or seltzer

     o Fresh fruit or herbs for flavor

     o Zevia soda (the orange flavor pairs wonderfully with tequila or vodka)

     o Stevia drops, like Hazelnut Liquid Stevia, which my husband enjoys adding to his whiskey.

   - Take Notes: Keep track of how different drinks affect you.

     o Does beer leave you feeling bloated?

     o Does Cabernet Sauvignon cause the scale to creep up or give you a headache?

     o Does Champagne work better for you than Prosecco?

Everyone's body reacts differently; this experimentation will help you make informed choices.

6. **Stick to One Drink**:

   - Start with a single serving:

   - One shot of liquor

   - 5-7 ounces of wine

- One beer or glass of bubbly

This is about enjoying the drink, not overindulging. Remember, a hangover is never fun, especially as we get older. And let's be honest, recovering from a bad hangover in your 40s, 50s, or beyond feels like it takes days.

Tips by Alcohol Type

- **Liquor**: Choose clean liquors like vodka, tequila, or whiskey, and add simple mixers like club soda or a splash of citrus. Avoid sugary cocktails like margaritas or daiquiris.

- **Beer**: If beer is your drink of choice, try light beer as a lower-calorie alternative. Save the heavier, more indulgent beers (like Guinness or craft IPAs) for special occasions as part of your 20% flexibility.

- **Wine**: Experiment with red and white wines to see what works best for your body. For example, you might find Merlot sits fine with you, while Chardonnay causes bloating or a headache.

- **Bubbly**: Champagne, Prosecco, and sparkling wines can vary widely in sugar content. Pay attention to how you feel after trying different brands or types. I prefer Cava from Spain. It generally has less sugar than the Italian Prosecco (and almost always costs less).

A Final Note

If you're someone who thinks, "I never get hangovers," please remember this: your body is now in a healthier, more balanced state. Drinking like you used to can hit you harder than you expect, so start slow and be mindful.

Taking a break from alcohol, whether it's for 30 days, six months, or even just a few weeks each year, can reset your body and your habits. You'll be surprised at how much clearer and more focused you feel, and you might even find that alcohol doesn't hold the same appeal as it once did.

Cheers to your health, balance, and success!

You Are a Warrior — Your Journey Is Real!

ProTip: Taking a break from alcohol doesn't mean giving up on fun. Recreate the experience with non-alcoholic drinks in your favorite glassware, yes, the stemmed one! Bring Zevia, or seltzer with you to a party. You can also get some root beer or cola flavored liquid Stevia and pour it over seltzer as a refreshing drink. Keep reminding yourself: this isn't forever, just for now. Your body will thank you for the reset. And when you're ready to reintroduce alcohol, treat it as a new experiment, one sip at a time. Cheers to progress, not perfection!

You Are a Warrior — Your Journey Is Real!

My Journey

If you believe giving up alcohol for 30 days will be difficult, what specifically are the challenges you are concerned about?

How has taking a break from alcohol impacted your body, mindset, or daily habits?

What new rituals or alternatives have you discovered that bring you the same sense of relaxation or enjoyment without alcohol?

_____

_____

_____

_____

_____

_____

_____

_____

_____

_____

_____

_____

CHAPTER 12

Sit on Your Hands (snacking)

"The best way to not feel hopeless is to get up and do something. Don't wait for good things to happen to you. If you go out and make some good things happen, you will fill the world with hope; you will fill yourself with hope."
— Barack Obama

Have you ever sat in front of your television and consumed handful after handful of chips, nuts, or popcorn? What about at the movies? I used to find it so difficult to go to the theater and not grab a large bucket of popcorn, no butter, but still! What is it about these moments that makes us forget our goals and eat, even when we're not hungry?

I believe a lot of it comes down to the movement of hand to mouth. That repetitive motion becomes automatic, almost meditative. We're not eating because we're hungry; we're eating because it's a habit, a reflex. Would you really eat as much if you stopped and counted each piece of popcorn, chip, or nut? Probably not, but really, who is going to count each kernel during a movie?

Our hands, mouth, and brain seem to act independently in these situations. I can't tell you how many times I've gone to a movie theater after a satisfying dinner and still consumed a giant tub of popcorn. My stomach doesn't need it, my brain knows it's unnecessary, and yet, my hands and mouth just keep going.

I've had countless clients tell me the same thing. Whether they're watching TV, reading, paying bills, or listening to music, they can easily consume an entire bag of chips, a bowl of nuts, or a large serving of popcorn without even realizing it.

It's time to acknowledge that our hands seem to have a mind of their own in these situations. So, let's outsmart them!

Give Your Hands Something To Do

If the hand-to-mouth habit is automatic, keeping your hands busy with something else is key. Here are some suggestions:

- Hold your book with both hands. It's tough to snack if your hands are occupied.

- Take up knitting or crocheting. I've had clients do this, and they've been amazed at how much it curbed their snacking.

- Scroll through your phone. Yes, we're told to put our phones down, but if using it keeps you from mindless eating, it's worth it.

- Polish your nails. You're not going to reach for snacks when your nails are wet!

- Give yourself a pedicure. Same idea, plus you'll have fabulous-looking toes.

- In your Balanced Warrior 30-Day Journal [https://30toLife.org], reflecting on your day or setting intentions is calming and productive.

- Work on your computer. Whether you're responding to emails, organizing your digital photos, or writing a to-do list, it's a great way to engage your hands and mind.

Keep Healthy Snacks Ready

Sometimes, the urge to snack isn't just about hand-to-mouth movement; it's a genuine craving for something to eat. That's okay! Just make sure you're prepared with healthier options. Always have something in the fridge that you can grab quickly and eat without guilt. Start by having a glass of water. Wait 15 minutes and see if you still have an urge to eat.

If you do, cold veggies are excellent for mindless snacking. They're low in calories, high in fiber, and satisfy the need for something crunchy. Here are some great options to keep on hand:

- Broccoli

- Cauliflower

- Carrots

- Green beans

- Cucumbers

- Cherry tomatoes

- Zucchini

- Asparagus

Steam them ahead of time or enjoy them raw. Either way, they're a fantastic go-to snack when the urge strikes.

If you're craving fruit, keep it to two servings daily. Fruits like blueberries, strawberries, cantaloupe, and honeydew are great choices, but they're easier to overeat than veggies. Grapes, for example, are high in sugar and can be addictive. I recommend limiting yourself to about 15 grapes per serving. You heard me, 15 grapes per serving. Any more than that can raise your glucose levels, which leads to extra sugar turning into fat, making it harder for your body to stay healthy and energized.

The beauty of non-starchy vegetables is that you can eat as much as you want. So, make those your primary snack option whenever possible. A short list of non-starchy vegetables can be found in your Balanced Warrior 30-Day Journal. Keep it on hand until you have memorized the list, making it easier to maintain your Freedom Eater 80/20 lifestyle.

Use Self-Hypnosis

Your self-hypnosis practice can be a powerful tool to curb mindless snacking. Spend 2–3 minutes reinforcing your commitment to your new healthy lifestyle. Visualize yourself feeling in control, making smart choices, and enjoying the benefits of your new habits. This small practice can shift your mindset and make a big difference.

Get Up and Move

If snacking is tied to sitting still for too long, break the cycle by getting up and moving your body. Here are a few quick ways to interrupt the urge:

- Take a walk around the room during TV commercials.
- Put in a load of laundry.
- Empty the dishwasher.

- Wipe down the stove (this is one of my go-to activities, it's the least I can do since I'm not the cook in our house).

Not only will this keep your hands busy, but you'll also get the added benefit of physical activity. Moving your body, even for a few minutes, can help reduce cravings and shift your focus away from food.

The Bottom Line

Mindless snacking is a habit; like any habit, it can be replaced with healthier behaviors. Keep your hands busy, drink a glass of water, prepare healthy snacks in advance, use your self-hypnosis, and get up and move when the urge strikes. These small changes will help you stay on track and feel more in control.

And remember, this is a journey. Each day presents an opportunity to learn more about yourself and cultivate a healthy, balanced lifestyle that suits you.

You Are a Warrior — Your Journey Is Real!

ProTip: Pay attention to when the urge to snack hits you. For many of my clients who work from home, 3:00 pm is a time when they get up, go to frig, and look for something. This is a habit I worked hard to replace. Now, I always have leftover cold non-starchy vegetables in the frig. My go-to for snacking is cold steamed broccoli, cauliflower, carrots, and green beans. This can be related to all of us coming home from school in the afternoon and having snacks. Notice when the urge strikes you. What else is going on?

You Are a Warrior — Your Journey Is Real!

My Journey

Think about the moments when you acted impulsively, what triggered those decisions, and how they made you feel afterward. Now, write down one or two strategies you will use to pause, reflect, and make a more mindful choice next time.

_____

_____

_____

_____

_____

_____

_____

_____

_____

_____

_____

_____

_____

CHAPTER 13

To Organic or Not to Organic

Grocery shopping today presents us with an array of choices. Labels like "Natural," "Grass-Fed," "Organic," "Hormone-Free," "Farm-Raised," and "Wild-Caught" can make things feel more complicated than they need to be. Ultimately, these choices come down to personal preference and budget. Here are a few practical tips to help you navigate these options.

Key Recommendations:

1. **Meat**: Avoid hormones in any meat products you purchase. This is one area where I strongly recommend investing. Hormone-free or grass-fed options are best when available and within your budget. Organic is great if you can find it and afford it.

2. **Fish**: Wild-caught fish is the healthier choice, though it's not always available and can be expensive. If you shop at Costco, check their freezer section for frozen wild-caught fish and shrimp; these can be more affordable. We buy the shrimp all the time.

3. **Rotisserie Chickens**: During the first 30 days, skip Costco's (or anyone else's) rotisserie chickens. Just trust me on this. Costco lists sugar on the ingredients and many other items. If you want to include rotisserie chicken, Whole Foods (check for a health food grocery in your area) makes an organic one. It's pricey but doesn't contain added ingredients to mess up your Balanced Warrior 30-day hormone balancing. If you find a local store that makes organic rotisserie chickens, be sure to check the ingredients.

4. **Deli Meat**: opt for low-sodium deli meat whenever possible.

Fruits and Vegetables: Organic or Not?

- If you eat a whole fruit or vegetable (e.g., apples, strawberries), buying organic is a good idea, as these items are more likely to carry pesticide residue. I recommend spending the extra on organic for all types of berries.

- If you don't eat the outside, such as with oranges or bananas, organic isn't as critical.

- With vegetables, it's a bit trickier. Many contain pesticides, so do your best to buy organic when possible. Local health food stores, seasonal farmers' markets, and larger chains like Whole Foods, Costco, and Trader Joe's often have organic options. However, organic produce tends to be more expensive, so weigh the cost against your priorities. For me, it's about balancing availability, convenience, cost, and supporting local stores. Do your best, but don't make yourself stressed or go broke trying to buy everything organic.

  ProTip: When choosing organic products, focus on the items that matter most. If budget constraints make buying all organic impractical, prioritize hormone-free meats, wild-caught fish, and organic produce for fruits and vegetables you consume whole, like berries or apples. Conventional options are typically fine for items with a peel, such as bananas or oranges. Balance is key, invest where it counts, and remember, every step toward healthier choices is progress.

ProTip 2: If you have Amazon Prime, you receive a discount at Whole Foods. If you pay with an Amazon Visa, you also get Amazon points when you shop at Whole Foods. I am not promoting Amazon, Whole Foods, or credit cards, but many clients have responded with, "Thanks, I never knew that."

You Are a Warrior — Your Journey Is Real!

My Journey

What's your approach to grocery shopping? Reflect on how you can make healthier food choices within your budget and lifestyle.

_____

_____

_____

_____

_____

_____

_____

_____

_____

_____

_____

_____

_____

_____

CHAPTER 14

The Art of Label Reading

"Let food be thy medicine and medicine be thy food"
— widely attributed to Hippocrates

Understanding food labels is one of the most important skills you can develop when trying to make healthier choices. My clients often hear me say: "If you can't pronounce it, you probably don't want to eat it." It's a good general rule.

In Chapter 27 on vitamins, I dive into label reading for supplements. Here, let's focus on food labels and some common traps consumers fall into.

The Myth of "All Natural"

Have you ever picked up a product that proudly declares itself "All Natural" and thought, "This must be good for me"? Let's take a closer look at various definitions used for the words "All Natural":

- **No Standard Definition**: In the U.S., the FDA has not set a strict definition for the term "All Natural." Generally, it means the product doesn't contain artificial flavors, colors, or synthetic substances. However, it doesn't mean it's free of sugar, corn syrup, sodium, or saturated fats.

- **Not Organic**: "All Natural" is not the same as "Organic." Organic certification involves specific farming methods, including the absence of pesticides, genetic modification, and synthetic fertilizers, none of which are addressed by the "All Natural" label.

- **Processed Ingredients**: Products labeled "All Natural" can still contain processed ingredients like "Natural Flavors," a vague term that often refers to lab-created additives.

- **Farming and Animal Welfare**: The "All Natural" label does not guarantee any particular farming practices, animal treatment, or absence of pesticides.

The key takeaway? Don't rely solely on the words "All Natural" on a label as an indicator of quality or health. Always read the full ingredients list and check for additional information.

Practical Label Reading

One of my clients recently encountered a common problem while following my Balanced Warrior 30-day recommendations. She was preparing a dish that called for two tablespoons of tomato sauce. She told her husband to pick up a sauce at the store with no sugar. After three trips back and forth, she finally reached out to me for clarification. The issue? Tomatoes naturally contain sugar, so she needed a sauce with **no added** sugar. It's a small but important distinction.

This story illustrates the importance of reading labels carefully. Here are some tips to get you started:

1. **Watch for Added Sugars**: Look for labels that say, "no added sugar." Natural sugars (like those found in fruit or tomatoes) are fine.

2. **Sodium**: Many processed foods, especially deli meats and canned goods, are high in sodium. Choose low-sodium options when possible.

3. **Don't Be Fooled by the Front**: Marketing terms like "Low Fat," "No Carbs," or "All Natural" are designed to catch your attention, but they don't tell the whole story. Turn the package over and read the nutritional facts and ingredient list for the real details.

Moving Forward

Don't feel pressured to be perfect as you begin your Balanced Warrior 30-day journey to balance and health. If you've already stocked your pantry with less-than-ideal options, there's no need to throw them out unless you want to. Instead, commit to being more conscious about your purchases moving forward.

This doesn't mean you must only buy organic, or "pure" products. Focus on what's most important to you while balancing budget, convenience, and practicality. The goal is to become more aware of what you're eating and how marketing influences our decisions.

When you take the time to read food labels and make informed choices, you're empowering yourself to make healthier decisions without falling victim to clever advertising. Remember, this is your journey, and I'm here to guide you as you navigate it in the best way for you. You've got this!

ProTip: Regarding food labels, the back of the package tells the real story. It's not about how many calories, net carbs, or fat. Look at the entire ingredient list. Focus on simple, recognizable ingredients and avoid products with added sugars or artificial additives. Remember, terms like "All Natural" or "Low Fat" are marketing tools, not health guarantees. The more informed you are, the more empowered you'll feel in making choices that align with your goals.

You Are a Warrior — Your Journey Is Real!

My Journey

What have you learned about reading labels? Jot down any surprising discoveries and how you'll use this knowledge moving forward.

_____

_____

_____

_____

_____

_____

_____

_____

_____

_____

_____

_____

_____

_____

PART 4

SPECIFIC CHALLENGES?

CHAPTER 15

Detox is a Real Thing

"Things sweet to taste prove in digestion sour."
— Shakespeare, Richard II

Let's talk about detox because it's real and normal when transitioning to a healthier lifestyle. By removing (or "crowding out") certain foods and replacing them with nourishing, whole, healthy options, your body begins to clean itself out naturally. This means flushing out toxins that may have built up over time in your body, often stored in excess fat.

While detox is a good thing, it's not always comfortable. Sometimes, the release of these toxins can create temporary, not-so-pleasant symptoms. It's important to know that these symptoms are usually short-lived, often appearing during the first week of your journey. They signify that your body is recalibrating and heading toward a healthier state.

That said, detox symptoms can vary significantly from person to person, and not everyone will experience them. If you do, remember that they are temporary and manageable. Most importantly, if you feel truly unwell, always reach out to your healthcare professional to rule out other potential issues.

Common Detox Symptoms

Here are some of the most common detox symptoms reported by clients, along with tips to manage them:

1. **Headaches**

   - Why it happens: Headaches are very common when reducing or eliminating caffeine. If you're used to drinking several cups of coffee or tea daily and have cut back to one caffeinated beverage daily, your body may be experiencing withdrawal from its usual caffeine levels.

   - How to manage it: Stay hydrated - drink plenty of water throughout the day. You are welcome to drink decaf coffee throughout the day. I would make a pot of decaf after my morning caffeinated cup, and it really helped me throughout the day, especially in the first couple of weeks. You can add some liquid-flavored Stevia to the decaf, and it will also give it a slightly sweet taste if that is something you crave.

   - The headaches usually pass within a day or two.

2. **Fatigue**

   - Why it happens: Your body is working hard to adjust to your new eating habits and is releasing stored toxins. This can leave you feeling more tired than usual.

- How to manage it: Honor your body's need for rest. Go to bed a little earlier, take short naps if possible, and avoid overexerting yourself. If your energy levels dip, focus on nutrient-dense meals and lighten your activity. Remember, during the Balanced Warrior 30-day balancing, you are avoiding intense workouts.

You are allowing your cortisol levels to balance.

3. **Constipation**

- Why it happens: Changes in your diet, especially if you increase your fiber intake from vegetables and other whole foods, can cause temporary digestive shifts.

- How to manage it: Stay hydrated (water is key) and try natural remedies like Smooth Move Tea or other gentle options. Be cautious with teas containing senna, as they can be strong for some people. Start by steeping the tea for just a few minutes to see how your body reacts. My clients find that any constipation goes away by the end of the Balanced Warrior 30-day balancing, and that it is manageable. If you are finding it challenging, you can also add (in very small amounts) more natural fiber to your diet through foods like flaxseeds, chia seeds, or prunes, or consult your healthcare provider about other gentle solutions.

4. **Flu-like Symptoms**

- Why it happens: Some clients reported feeling like they have the flu, with symptoms like mild aches, chills, or a general "blah" feeling. If you experience this, it may be that your body is shedding unnecessary toxins and adjusting to the cleaner foods you're eating.

- How to manage it: Focus on rest, hydration, and warm, soothing meals like broths or teas. These symptoms typically clear up within a few days. However, if they persist or worsen, check in with your healthcare provider to ensure there's nothing more serious going on.

Other Potential Symptoms

Here are a few additional, less common symptoms that can appear during detox:

- **Mood swings or irritability**: Your mood may fluctuate as your body adjusts to changes in sugar, caffeine, and processed food intake. Breathe, hydrate, and remind yourself that this will pass.

- **Skin breakouts**: Your skin is an elimination organ, so some people notice minor breakouts or increased oiliness during detox. Stick with your skincare routine, drink water, and let it run its course. Be mindful of using body lotions with a lot of oil. You are cleaning out fats such as oils. Use a small amount or skip the body lotion for 30 days, if you can.

- **Cravings**: Your body may crave the very foods you're trying to remove (like sugar or processed snacks). Use this as an opportunity to explore healthier alternatives and remind yourself why you're making these changes.

The Bigger Picture

Detox is a temporary process, and the symptoms, if they appear, are a sign that your body is recalibrating and moving toward better health. The key is to stay patient, kind, and understanding with yourself during this time.

Here are some general tips to help ease the detox process:

- **Hydrate**: Drink plenty of water to help your body flush out toxins. Herbal teas and broths can also be soothing and hydrating.

- **Eat nutrient-dense foods**: Focus on whole, unprocessed foods like leafy greens, colorful vegetables, lean proteins, and healthy fats to support your body's detoxification process.

- **Rest**: Listen to your body's needs and give it the rest it requires to adjust to these changes.

- **Stay positive**: Remember that these symptoms are temporary and part of a positive transformation. Soon, you'll feel more energetic, lighter, and healthier. You have committed yourself. Detox is a minor; short-lived inconvenience compared with the gift of "thinness" and health you are gaining.

A Final Thought

Detoxing isn't just about removing toxins; it's about replacing negative habits with positive ones. By crowding out processed, unhealthy foods with nourishing, whole foods, you're giving yourself a fresh start.

You'll notice a remarkable shift in just a few days as the symptoms pass. Many clients report feeling clearer, more energized, and just plain better. This process is a gift you're giving yourself, so trust the journey and know that the rewards will come soon enough.

You Are a Warrior — Your Journey Is Real!

ProTip: Detox is your body's way of saying, "Thanks for giving me a break!" Remember, hydration is your best friend during this phase. Try keeping a water bottle close by and infusing it with slices of lemon or cucumber for a refreshing twist. Don't forget this is temporary, and every symptom is a sign that your body is adjusting and moving toward balance. A warm cup of herbal tea or a quick walk can do wonders to ease discomfort. You're clearing out the old to make way for the new.

You Are a Warrior — Your Journey Is Real!

My Journey

What physical or emotional detox symptoms have you experienced in the past? Write about how you can stay kind to yourself during this part of the process.

_____

_____

_____

_____

_____

_____

_____

_____

_____

_____

_____

_____

_____

_____

_____

CHAPTER 16

Two Steps Forward, One Step Back

"Our greatest glory is not in never falling, but in rising every time we fall." — Confucius

---

Once you begin your Balanced Warrior 30-day balancing, most mornings will start with a smile as you step on the scale. Whether the number reflects a steady downward trend or a gradual pattern unique to your body, you'll notice progress. However, there may be days when the scale doesn't move, or even shows a small gain.

This can happen for many reasons:

- A bit of extra salt in your meals

- Not getting in all your water (you need to drink half your body weight in ounces of water every day, up to 100 ounces)

- Skipping meals or not eating enough food

- Constipation or irregular digestion

- Hormonal changes like your period

- Or even the result of a small deviation from the Balanced Warrior 30-day plan

Oh no! Did I just say you might stray a bit? Let's address this head-on right now.

Acknowledging the Journey

I invite you to embrace this truth and incorporate this as one of your new life's mantras: "I am creating a new, healthy lifestyle."

This isn't about perfection; it's about progress. You're finally replacing habits that no longer serve you and learning what it feels like to take control of your body, your mind, and your relationship with food.

But replacing habits is NEVER a straight path.

Even with the best of intentions, life will happen. You might go to a party, attend a birthday celebration, enjoy a dinner date, or face an unexpected social situation. In moments like these, you may feel like deviating from the plan. And guess what? That's okay.

Most of my clients experience these moments. It took me seven months to reach my Ideal Healthy Weight. During those months, I deviated on Thanksgiving. It's a favorite meal of mine, and I wanted to enjoy it. And when the scale reflects something unexpected, like a gain or stagnation, many respond with newfound strength.

One woman told me, "It doesn't bother me anymore. I know my body is getting healthier every day. The scale will move down again." She went on to release 35 pounds and has kept it off for three years.

You see, the key isn't avoiding those moments. Learning how to respond to them without guilt, shame, or frustration is the key.

The One Absolute

The one non-negotiable in this journey?

Weigh yourself every single day. Yes, even on days when you feel like you've gone off course.

One of the toughest moments can be stepping on the scale the day after you strayed and seeing a higher number. It might sting, but know this:

It's temporary.

This is your opportunity to learn about your body. To discover patterns. To understand what works and what doesn't. This journey isn't about punishing yourself for perceived "failures." It's about replacing old, unhelpful habits with ones that will serve you for the rest of your life.

So, if the scale goes up, jump right back into the process.

You Are a Warrior — Your Journey Is Real!

Your Emotional Toolkit

Let's talk about those negative emotions — guilt, shame, and frustration- that might creep in during this process. These emotions no longer have a seat at your table. You're in control now.

But let's be real: they might still show up uninvited from time to time. Even I still wrestle with fleeting moments of self-doubt or frustration, and I have been living this lifestyle since 2021.

So, what can you do?

Find the feelings that do serve you. Replace negativity with feelings of:

- Control (you're steering your ship)

- Pride (look how far you've come!)

- Joy (you're changing your life)

- Excitement (you're on a journey to freedom)

What works for you? Maybe it's putting reminders by your scale, positive affirmations, pictures, or words that instantly shift your mindset. Maybe it's self-hypnosis, meditation, a walk in nature, or some yoga. Whatever grounds you and re-centers your focus, make it a part of your toolkit.

Breaking the Pattern

It's important to recognize that you didn't gain weight, develop sugar or salt cravings, or turn to food for comfort all in one day. These patterns developed over the years, even decades.

Now, you're stopping the cycle. You're breaking free from the madness of yo-yo dieting. You're learning how to live diet-free.

And that's why small setbacks won't derail you. Because this isn't a diet, it's a lifestyle. Every single step forward, no matter how small, brings you closer to a lifetime of health, freedom, and balance.

Two steps forward, one step back? That's still one step ahead.

Final Thoughts

This journey is about YOU, your body, your mindset, and your choices. It's not about perfection; it's about showing up for yourself every day.

Remember that you are in control when you wake up tomorrow, no matter what the scale says.

You're creating a new life, one habit at a time. Celebrate every step forward, learn from every step back, and keep moving toward the life you deserve.

You Are a Warrior — Your Journey Is Real!

ProTip: Progress isn't linear, and that's okay! Every step forward, no matter how small, counts towards your goals. Keep writing your small victories in your Balanced Warrior 30-Day Journal (don't forget your non-scale victories), whether it's mastering a new recipe or staying on track with water intake. I know; keeping a journal keeps coming up. Why? Because journaling reinforces your commitment to your goals. You can also talk to your phone if that is easier than writing. Right now, we can ask Siri (or Gemini or Google) to take a Note for us. If the scale stops moving, focus on how your clothes fit, energy levels, or other non-scale victories. And remember, two steps forward and one step back is still a step ahead!

You Are a Warrior — Your Journey Is Real!

My Journey

How do you typically handle setbacks? Write about reframing "slips" as part of the process and committing to progress over perfection.

_____

_____

_____

_____

_____

_____

_____

_____

_____

_____

_____

_____

_____

_____

_____

_____

CHAPTER 17

Oh No! Down the Rabbit Hole (and Meeting Your Self-Saboteur)

Alice: *"Would you tell me, please, which way I ought to go from here?"*

The Cheshire Cat: *"That depends a good deal on where you want to get to."*

Alice: *"I don't much care where—"*

The Cheshire Cat: *"Then it doesn't matter which way you go."*

— Lewis Carroll, *Alice's Adventures in Wonderland*

How many times have you been fully committed to your health and weight loss goals, only to find yourself inexplicably tumbling down the rabbit hole? It's a familiar scenario. You wake up feeling absolutely determined to stick to your plan. The day starts off great.

You're motivated, have prepared your meals, and feel confident about your progress.

Then, it happens. You arrive at work, and someone (how dare they) has brought donuts to the office. Or maybe it's bagels, cookies, or a homemade cake.

At first, you resist. You tell yourself, "Nope, I've got this. I've been so good." But then, something switches. A little voice whispers, "Go ahead, just one piece won't hurt. You've earned it." Before you know it, your hand reaches for the donut, and you're savoring every bite.

What happened? How did your resolve melt away in a matter of seconds?

Recognizing the Role of Self-Sabotage

Here's the truth: we all have an inner self-saboteur waiting for just the right moment to strike. That saboteur is often the unseen force dragging you down the rabbit hole. It's the voice in your head that nudges you when you're tired, hungry, bored, upset, nervous, or even happy.

It's the part of you that says:

- "You've been so good—why not treat yourself?"
- "You're having such a tough day; you deserve this."
- "You forgot to bring lunch today—it's not your fault, so go ahead and indulge." Sound familiar?

But something important to know is that your self-saboteur isn't trying to ruin your life. It's coming from a place of wanting to make you comfortable.

If you've historically turned to food for comfort, your saboteur sees that as a quick fix to make you feel better. If sweets have always made you happy, your saboteur will push you toward the chocolate cake. If salty snacks are your go-to, it'll convince you that one potato chip won't hurt.

The challenge is that the "comfort" your saboteur offers is fleeting. That donut or bag of chips might feel great for 10 seconds, but the spiral of guilt, self-judgment, and frustration that follows can undo the progress you've made, and even worse, it can leave you doubting yourself.

Meeting Your Saboteur

Recognizing and confronting your saboteur is one of the most powerful tools to break free from self-sabotage.

Take a moment to visualize it. What does your self-saboteur look like? Stand in front of a mirror and imagine it sitting on your shoulder. Is it a tiny devil with a mischievous grin? A shadowy figure? A younger version of yourself?

Once you have that image in mind, talk to your saboteur.

- **Acknowledge it**: Thank it for trying to protect you or comfort you.

- **Set boundaries**: Let your saboteur know that YOU are in control and that while you appreciate its input, now isn't the time.

- **Reframe the moment**: Remind your saboteur that you're not saying you'll NEVER have that food again. You're simply choosing not to have it right now because you're focused on your goal.

This isn't about fighting your saboteur. It's about building a relationship with it and understanding its intentions, so you can make conscious choices rather than reacting impulsively. The Rabbit Hole Spiral

Here's where self-sabotage and the rabbit hole collide:

Once you've given in to temptation, whether it's a donut, a piece of cake, or French fries, it's easy to feel like the day is ruined. You think, "I've already messed up, so what's the point? I'll start again tomorrow."

This is when self-judgment takes over, and it can be brutal. You beat yourself up for slipping, and that harsh inner critic only fuels the downward spiral. One "off-plan" moment turns into an entire day (or weekend) of poor choices, leaving you feeling defeated and stuck.

Breaking Free: What Would Happen If You Didn't Spiral?

Here's a question: What if you didn't go down the rabbit hole?

What if, instead of letting one slip-up define your entire day, you permitted yourself to enjoy the indulgence and then moved on?

Let's say you have the donut. What if you savored and appreciated it and then returned to your plan immediately afterward?

You don't have to wait until tomorrow to get back on track. In fact, the faster you reset, the more empowered you'll feel. Remember, your day is never based on what you do or don't eat, it's about how you respond and what you accomplish overall.

Practical Tools to Regain Control

Here are some actionable steps to help you navigate temptation and avoid spiraling:

1. **Pause Before You Indulge**: The next time you're confronted with a tempting food, pause for 30 minutes.

During that time:

- Drink water, herbal tea, or coffee. o Distract yourself with a task or activity.

- Reflect on whether you're truly hungry or just reacting to emotion.

If you still want the food after 30 minutes, go ahead and enjoy it, guilt-free.

2. **Visualize Your Saboteur**: Picture your saboteur and address it directly. Acknowledge its intentions but remind it that you're in control.

3. **Use Self-Hypnosis**: Take 5 minutes to do a self-hypnosis exercise. Reconnect with your goals, reinforce your motivation, and remind yourself of your why. You can do this in your car or the Ladies' Room.

4. **Shift Your Focus**: List everything you accomplished that day, big or small. This practice can help you see the bigger picture and shift your focus away from food.

5. **Repeat Your Why**: Write your why 20 times on paper, say it out loud, or type it on your phone. Keep it front and center to remind yourself of the deeper reason you're on this journey.

Final Thoughts

Self-sabotage and the rabbit hole go hand in hand, but they don't have to control your story. You can take back control and stay on track by recognizing your saboteur, reframing slip-ups, and using the tools available.

Remember: one choice does not define your day, week, or journey. You're allowed to step backward for a moment; sometimes sh*t happens. I can tell you that YOU ARE ALWAYS IN CONTROL, AND CAN PREVENT A SLIPUP, but the truth is, it does happen. Don't stress. Move your mind away from recrimination and guilt. That's how you avoid going down that rabbit hole versus just looking down it.

You deserve to reach your Ideal Healthy Weight, to feel good, and to live a life that brings you joy. And you can do that without letting a donut or your saboteur take the wheel. You are now armed with ways to deal with your saboteur.

You Are a Warrior — Your Journey Is Real!

ProTip: Your self-saboteur thrives on impulse, but you hold the power to pause and reset. Visualize your saboteur as a quirky character, give it a name, a voice, or a costume! When temptation strikes, acknowledge it with humor: "Nice try, Debbie the Donut Diva, but I'm in charge today!" Pair this mental exercise with a simple action, like drinking a glass of water or taking three deep breaths, to regain control. Remember, one choice doesn't define your journey; you do.

You Are a Warrior — Your Journey Is Real!

My Journey

What triggers your self-sabotaging behaviors? Reflect on how you can identify and manage those moments when they arise. List three actions you can take to gain back control.

_____

_____

_____

_____

_____

_____

_____

_____

_____

_____

_____

_____

_____

_____

CHAPTER 18

Never Say Never
(and Know Your Limits)

"If you obey all the rules, you miss all the fun."
–Katharine Hepburn

One of my core beliefs is that no food should be a "never have." I'm not referring to foods you avoid for allergies, sensitivities, religious customs, or similar reasons. I'm talking about the idea that to maintain your Ideal Healthy Weight (IHW), you must absolutely, forever, avoid the foods you love.

Some may disagree with me, and that's okay. But here's my reasoning: our subconscious minds don't respond well to the word "never." If you've ever told a two-year-old or a teenager they can never do something, you already know what happens next, they immediately want to do it more!

Teenagers are masters of this game. When my son was younger, we would let him join us at holiday dinners with a small taste of wine. Some people thought I was out of my mind, but my perspective was simple: anything that feels forbidden often becomes more tempting. Of course, this is just my personal experience, but it's a lesson that stuck with me.

If I were to tell you that you can never have ice cream, chocolate, cotton candy, or a Big Mac ever again, your subconscious would likely rebel. For many of us, it's less about the food and more about independence and personal choice. Being told "no" often makes us crave that thing even more.

Instead, I want to teach you how to enjoy the foods you love occasionally and mindfully. One important caveat: if you know certain foods trigger uncontrollable cravings, foods you can't stop eating once you start, we need to address those separately. I call these Trigger Foods, which brings us to the next section.

Trigger Foods – The Ones You Can't Have Just One Of

If you've ever seen me at a party, you'll likely find me standing by the shrimp or the cashews. These are two of my Trigger Foods I can't stop eating once I start. Shrimp frequently appear in my husband's giant salads, and he still weighs out our portions to keep me in check. As for cashews, they're never in my house unless I'm hosting company, and even then, I know I'll eat more than my guests. Whatever's left goes home with someone else, no exceptions.

Do you remember the old Lays Potato Chips slogan, "Bet you can't eat just one"? That sums up my relationship with tortilla chips. The only time I allow myself to indulge is at a Mexican restaurant, where the temptation is unavoidable but contained.

Another big one for me? French fries. If someone at the table orders them, I will pick at them. Once I start, it's hard to stop.

Recognizing and Managing Trigger Foods

We all have foods that override our ability to stop eating, even when we're not hungry. The first and most crucial step is to recognize which foods fall into this category for you. My top suggestion? Don't buy them.

Clients often ask, "But what if other people in my household love those foods?" Here's the solution: let them store it somewhere you won't see or reach it. Out of sight, out of mind. I can't explain the exact psychological reason for this mindless eating behavior, but I know that staying away from these foods is key unless they're portioned out in advance.

For example, buy single-serving portions instead of buying a big jar of cashews or a family-sized bag of chips. I will buy the one-ounce portion bags of almonds that Trader Joe's carries. This way, you're more in control.

I confess that if we have friends over, I may buy a big-sized fancy mixed nuts. Yup, they have cashews. And, yes, I am the one you must stop from picking out all the cashews. In this scenario, I allow myself to indulge and then send the rest of the nuts home with my visitors. They cannot stay in my house.

Navigating Social Settings and Trigger Foods

The challenge gets trickier when people bring these foods into your home or when you're at a party or holiday gathering.

Here's what I recommend:

- If someone brings trigger foods to your home, thank them graciously and send them home with the leftovers.

- If leftovers can't go home with someone, throw them away. Yes, I said it. Throw. Them. Away. While it might feel wasteful (and you might hear that voice saying, "But there are starving people somewhere"), remind yourself that eating the leftovers won't help anyone. Instead, it will likely derail your progress and worsen your mental and physical health.

What about freezing trigger foods? It's not a foolproof solution. If you've ever defrosted a cookie, cake, or bagel in the microwave for 15 seconds because you had to have it right then and there, you know what I mean. A friend once joked, "The only freezer that works is someone else's!" And she's right.

Planning Ahead

Dining out or eating at someone else's home adds another layer of complexity, but planning makes all the difference.

- **At a friend's house**: If you're comfortable, ask your host what's on the menu and share your preferences. Most people are understanding, especially when it comes to dietary restrictions.

- **At a restaurant**: Look at the menu online ahead of time and decide what you'll order before you even arrive. Many restaurants are willing to accommodate dietary preferences, so don't hesitate to ask for adjustments. For example, I always tell servers that I avoid dairy. It's not an allergy, just a preference, but they're usually happy to help.

Using Self-Hypnosis to Tackle Trigger Foods

One of the most powerful tools you can use is self-hypnosis. This technique can help you retrain your subconscious mind to feel full, satisfied, and happy after eating just one cookie, one piece of chocolate, or one small handful of cashews. By replacing unwanted habits with positive ones, you can take control of your relationship with food and enjoy the occasional indulgence without going overboard.

You Are a Warrior — Your Journey Is Real!

ProTip: Trigger foods don't have to control you. Recognize your patterns and plan ahead. If you know you can't resist tortilla chips or cashews, create boundaries, like only enjoying them in single servings or at specific occasions. Remember, it's okay to send your guests home with leftover "trigger" foods, and it's OK to throw them out. Out of sight, truly, is out of mind! Use self-hypnosis to reinforce your confidence in enjoying indulgences without overindulging. And remember, enjoying food mindfully is about freedom, not restriction.

You Are a Warrior — Your Journey Is Real!

My Journey

What foods or habits feel off-limits for you? Write about how you can create balance by enjoying what you love in moderation.

_____

_____

_____

_____

_____

_____

_____

_____

_____

_____

_____

_____

_____

CHAPTER 19

Making Comparisons

"I'll have what she's having." — Random Diner
Customer, *When Harry Met Sally*

While having what Sally had that day for lunch may be a comparison that still makes us smile, comparing yourself to anyone else can be another trip down that rabbit hole.

I remember hearing this question as a kid: "Who would you rather be?" I don't know precisely who would ask this, a close friend, a teacher, or maybe something I read or saw on television. But I distinctly recall that no matter how miserable I might have been then, my answer was always the same: there is no one I'd rather be.

That doesn't mean I didn't cry myself to sleep wishing I wasn't fat, wishing my skin would clear up, or hoping that some boy would like me. Those feelings were very real, and they hurt. But somewhere deep inside, I knew I didn't want to become someone else, not a particular movie star, not the teacher's pet, not even one of the "thin" girls who seemed to have it all together.

Looking back, I realize now that I must have intuitively understood, even as a child, that no one else's life is perfect. What challenges did they face? What heartaches or struggles were they hiding? What was their true story? Maybe it came down to that old saying: "Better the devil you know than the devil you don't."

That inner knowing at a young age didn't mean I was immune to comparing myself to others, far from it. As a kid, I was ridiculed for being overweight, and it was impossible not to notice the thin girls around me. The comparisons followed me through life, long after school days were behind me. As I shed weight, regained it, and went through the endless dieting cycles, I couldn't help but compare myself to the women I saw in restaurants, magazines, books, or on television. And yes, I still do it. But now, when those thoughts pop into my head, I've trained myself to dismiss them quickly.

These days, the comparisons look a little different. Sometimes, I think, "I wonder if she's older than me?" But as soon as I notice those thoughts, I practice releasing them. Because I know this truth: comparing yourself to others is always a no-win situation.

Stop Comparing; Start Noticing

Let me clarify something: I don't mean you should stop noticing people. Notice them! Appreciate them! Find something admirable about others, but don't compare yourself to them.

For me, noticing people often leads to compliments. And there's real magic in giving someone a genuine compliment. A simple "I love your nails" or "That color looks amazing on you" can light up someone's face with a smile. It's one of the easiest ways to spread kindness in the world.

ProTip: Accepting compliments is just as important as giving them. I'll admit, I still struggle with this. My reflex is to respond with a qualifier: "Oh, this old thing?" or "It's nothing special." But graciously accepting a compliment or gift is part of recognizing your value. You are unique. You brighten the lives of those around you just by being YOU.

Social Media and the Comparison Trap

Let's talk about one of the biggest culprits of comparison these days: social media. Between Facebook, Instagram, TikTok, and other platforms, you can easily spend hours scrolling and wondering:

- How does she look that amazing in every single photo or video?

- How does their life look so perfect?

- Why do they have more followers, likes, or comments than I?

- Are they using filters or editing their pictures?

It's easy to get lost in this maze. And here's the thing: it's not just about comparing appearances anymore. Social media has turned comparison into a competition for validation. You're only seeing the highlights of someone else's life, not the whole picture. In addition, filters are now used when taking a photo. I even have the Beauty APP on my phone that makes me look fabulous every time.

If you find yourself spiraling into the comparison trap, use your self-hypnosis to pull yourself out. Create a personalized affirmation, like: "I am unique. I have value. I spend my time focused on _____." Fill in that blank with something meaningful, whether spending quality time with loved ones, working on a project, or simply enjoying your own company.

129

Comparison in Weight-Release Journeys

Comparisons often creep up in weight-release programs, especially in group settings. It's common for couples, especially men and women, to do my program together. I'll tell you a secret: men almost always release weight faster. It's just biology.

I vividly recall one married couple who turned their Balanced Warrior 30-day balancing program into a friendly competition. They motivated each other by making it fun and stayed neck and neck the entire time. Ultimately, she reached her Ideal Healthy Weight (IHW) and has maintained it ever since.

Unfortunately, he didn't stick with the program long-term.

Here's the key takeaway: each person's journey is unique. It's not about how fast or slow someone else is progressing. What matters is staying consistent with your goals and your progress.

The Beauty of Your Path

I know it's tempting to compare your progress to someone else's. But the moment you do that, you lose sight of all the big and small victories unique to your path.

You'll notice how far you've come when you focus on your journey. You'll see your strength, resilience, and growth. And you'll realize that you are exactly where you're meant to be.

So, let go of the comparisons. Instead, celebrate who you are. Celebrate your progress. Celebrate that there's no one else in the world exactly like YOU.

You Are a Warrior — Your Journey Is Real!

ProTip: Comparing yourself to others is like measuring the ocean with a teaspoon, impossible and unnecessary! Focus instead on celebrating your unique journey. Replace comparisons with compliments; finding something kind to say about others will shift the energy and lift you both. Remember that when scrolling social media, you're seeing highlights, not the whole story. Create an affirmation like, "I am exactly where I need to be, and my progress is my own." Finally, turn envy into inspiration by asking, "What can I learn from this person that aligns with my goals?" Celebrate YOU, because there's no one else like you in this world.

You Are a Warrior — Your Journey Is Real!

My Journey

How often do you compare yourself to others? Take a moment to reflect on how comparisons have shaped your thoughts, actions, or feelings. Now, jot down one or two ways you can focus on your unique progress and celebrate your wins, big or small.

_____

_____

_____

_____

_____

_____

_____

_____

_____

_____

_____

_____

_____

_____

CHAPTER 20

Control in Chaos

"You just got lesson number one: don't think; it can only hurt the ball club." — Crash Davis, *Bull Durham*

As you continue to use self-hypnosis to give yourself powerful, positive suggestions, you will notice how much more in control you feel. This isn't just about food.

Let's face it, life often feels like a juggling act, where one wrong move sends everything crashing down. Whether it's work deadlines, family obligations, or the never-ending ping of notifications, the world seems designed to test our limits. And when life feels chaotic, what do we do? We cling to the one thing we think we can control.

For many women, that's food. Dieting offers the illusion of control. The strict rules, the calorie counts, the "good" and "bad" foods all feel like a system we can master. But here's the catch: that tight grip often leaves us cranky, exhausted, and more out of balance than ever.

I have found that sticking to a strict diet plan, while making me cranky, also made me feel more in control of my life. I could do anything if I could resist the temptation of the donuts and bagels at work. Remember, the subconscious is a powerful undercurrent that is always present and looking out for our best interests. Little kids know how to get control when they want something or feel overwhelmed; they cry.

We live in a world where we often feel out of control. Technology has made our lives easier, but not simpler. I have often felt like throwing my computer out the window when Zoom or some other application doesn't function correctly.

Control isn't about restriction; it's about awareness and alignment. It's not just what you eat; it's how you feel about it. When you start using tools like self-hypnosis, you'll discover that control isn't about perfection. It's about collaboration with your body, your subconscious, and even that inner four-year-old still throwing tantrums when life feels overwhelming.

Why Overwhelm Equals Out-of-Control

Feeling overwhelmed is a universal experience for women. We constantly shift between roles as we navigate careers, relationships, and family. One minute we're the boss in the boardroom; the next, we're the carpool driver, caring for elderly parents, watching grandchildren, paying bills, grocery shopping, or the chef in the kitchen (men in my life have all cooked. As my mother would remind me, necessity is the mother of invention). No wonder our self-talk can spiral into negativity.

Here's the kicker: Overwhelm feeds the subconscious belief that we're failing. And when we feel like we're failing, we grasp at control, sometimes in unhelpful ways. Whether mindlessly eating chips after a stressful day or diving headfirst into an overly restrictive diet, these behaviors are our subconscious trying to regain a sense of stability.

Reclaiming Control in a Healthy Way

This is where self-hypnosis shines. It's not just about food, it's about rewiring your inner dialogue to support you, rather than sabotage you. Imagine speaking to yourself with the same kindness and encouragement you'd offer your best friend. That's what self-hypnosis helps you achieve.

The power lies in small, consistent shifts:

- Recognizing when overwhelm is driving your choices.
- Redirecting your subconscious with positive suggestions.
- Aligning your actions with your actual goals rather than reactive habits.

When you learn to embrace these tools, you'll find that control isn't something you force but flow into. Suddenly, resisting the donuts at work isn't about white-knuckling willpower. It's about making a choice that aligns with the vibrant, healthy life you're creating.

Feeling in control is a significant part of your new, healthier lifestyle. Being conscious and aware of what you put in your mouth, understanding and working with your subconscious to be at your best, is a place many people never get to.

Your ability to use self-hypnosis, to understand and accept your four-year-old emotional self, and to collaborate with her to accomplish your goals is VERY POWERFUL STUFF.

Practice your self-hypnosis; when you feel ready, you can expand your suggestions to whatever you desire. (We dive into Self-hypnosis in Chapter 25.)

Most women I work with are professionals, business owners, or in the corporate world. In other words, they work outside the home. Maintaining a sense of control and balance between work and home is a challenge that women always discuss with me. Whether an entrepreneur or climbing the corporate ladder, feeling overwhelmed does not bode well for feeling in control. As women, we switch hats all the time. Our self-talk is often negative, and we are habitually our "own worst enemy." Your self-hypnosis can help you in any area of your life. It will allow you to eliminate being good on your diet with an overall sense of control in all areas of your life.

You Are a Warrior — Your Journey Is Real!

ProTip: Control doesn't come from rigid rules; it's built through small, consistent choices that align with your goals. When life feels chaotic, pause and redirect your energy toward positive actions. Work on getting into a calmer place before you are completely overwhelmed. Use tools like self-hypnosis to reset your mindset and focus on what truly matters. Remember, control isn't about doing everything perfectly but finding balance and flow amid the chaos. Whether saying no to donuts or setting boundaries with your time, every step forward is progress.

You Are a Warrior — Your Journey Is Real!

My Journey

What areas of your life feel out of control? Reflect on how finding balance in those areas might improve your relationship with food and health.

_____

_____

_____

_____

_____

_____

_____

_____

_____

_____

_____

_____

_____

PART 5

THE PLAN

CHAPTER 21

30-Day Balancing – Balanced Warrior — Phase One

"Diets or past failures will not defeat me. Instead, I choose balance and confidence." — Debbie Harris

---

Before we get started, I want you to know that the Balanced Warrior 30-day balancing is ONLY 30 days. After that, we will reintroduce other foods back into your life. As you progress through the Balanced Warrior, Harmony Heroine, and finally, Freedom Eater phases, you will reach your Ideal Healthy Weight and stay there easily and effortlessly.

The Balanced Warrior phase is where the magic begins. This is more than cutting out certain foods or reducing calories; it's about recalibrating your body's internal systems, especially hormones. By the end of these 30 days, you'll see changes on the scale and feel them in your energy levels, clarity of mind, and overall well-being.

Why Balancing Works

When we talk about weight and overall health, hormones play a significant role. Three key players we're focusing on are:

1. **Cortisol (the stress hormone)**: Elevated cortisol levels, whether from chronic stress, lack of sleep, or intense exercise, signal your body to hold onto fat, especially around the midsection. By eliminating sugars, unhealthy fats, processed foods, and starchy vegetables and focusing on nutrient-dense options, we help lower cortisol levels, allowing our bodies to release stored fat. While many cortisol-balancing programs eliminate caffeine entirely, you may enjoy one caffeinated beverage daily. It's 100% doable, and you're way more likely to stick to this new lifestyle forever and keep the weight off. You can continue to greet each morning with a nice hot mug of coffee or tea. Skip the urge to grab that afternoon mug, it'll be worth it. In a few days, you won't miss it. Soda, unless it's Zevia brand, is not permitted.

2. **Insulin (the storage hormone)**: Sugar and starch intake cause insulin to spike, leading to fat storage and energy crashes. Removing these foods during this phase helps stabilize insulin levels, which in turn improves fat loss and overall energy.

3. **Leptin and Ghrelin (the hunger hormones)**: Leptin tells your brain when you're full, and ghrelin signals hunger. Imbalances can make you feel ravenous or disconnected from natural hunger cues. Clean, whole foods help reset these signals, empowering you to regain control over your appetite.

This phase isn't just about weight release; it's a reset button for your entire body. You're giving yourself a chance to heal, recharge, and thrive. You'll notice clearer skin, better sleep, reduced brain fog, and increased energy.

Think of this phase as the foundation for your 80/20 Lifestyle, the Freedom Eater phase, where all of this is naturally incorporated into your new forever lifestyle. (Discussed in Chapter 24.) Whether you use medication or supplements alongside this program, balancing your hormones and nourishing your body and mind with the right foods will help create long-term success.

Getting Started: Loading Days and Supplies

Before diving into the Balanced Warrior phase, let's prepare! The first two days of this program are called loading or prep days. You'll eat anything you love for these two days, yes, you read that right. Indulge in your favorite foods and prepare your body for the journey ahead. One tip: stick with fats and starches. It is best, when loading, not to consume a bag of cookies, bars of candy, or any other high-sugar foods. Okay for some sugar, but don't make that your primary loading food.

Why Loading Days Matter

You might wonder, "Why on earth would I eat everything I love before I start this program?" Here's why:

1. Loading/prep days help ensure your body isn't in a "starvation" mode when you cut down on calories, sugar, and unhealthy fats. This lets your metabolism start strong and prevents an energy crash.

2. Psychologically, indulging for two days helps you feel ready to commit fully to the Balanced Warrior 30-day balancing

process. This isn't about deprivation, it's about resetting, learning, and creating a healthier lifestyle.

What to Enjoy on Loading Days: Here are some examples of what my clients have enjoyed:

- Pizza

- Pasta

- French fries

- Ice cream

- Sushi

- Baguette and brie (or your favorite cheese)

- Chocolate (Dark chocolate is best)

- Your favorite alcoholic beverages

The idea isn't to gorge yourself but to enjoy the foods you'll give up for 30 days. Eat until you're satisfied and focus on fats and starches rather than loading up on sugary desserts all day.

Supplies to Have on Hand

A little preparation goes a long way. Here's what you'll need:

- A digital food scale to weigh your proteins.

- A digital bathroom scale to track your daily progress.

- A good non-stick pan for cooking with minimal or no fat.

- Herbs and spices to add flavor (check labels to ensure no added sugar or salt).

- Sea or Celtic salt for seasoning.

- Liquid Stevia (plain or flavored). Avoid powdered sweeteners unless they are organic and solely Stevia-based.

- Zevia soda (Stevia-sweetened) for a guilt-free treat.

Getting Started

Congratulations! You're embarking on a 30-day health journey to literally "give your body a break." Inflammation will reduce, aches and pains may diminish, your sleep will improve, and weight and inches will release. Be sure to read Chapter 15 before you begin where we discuss the possibility of Detox symptoms.

Why Are We Eliminating These Foods?

Let's look at why removing sugar, alcohol, unhealthy fats, and starchy vegetables is so impactful:

1. **Sugar**: Reducing sugar intake balances blood sugar levels and improves insulin sensitivity. Processed sugar is hiding in so many of our foods, making it critical to remove during this phase.

2. **Alcohol**: Eliminating alcohol leads to better sleep and lower stress hormone levels, primarily cortisol. Sleep plays a huge role in balancing hormones.

3. **Starchy Vegetables**: Avoiding potatoes, corn, peas, and winter squash helps stabilize blood sugar and prevent insulin spikes, keeping your hormones balanced.

4. **Caffeine**: Limiting caffeine to one cup daily supports balanced cortisol and stress regulation. You still get the boost without overloading your system.

(Citations for these points are included on the website's References page at https://30toLife.org/References.)

What You'll Be Eating Daily:

Here's what your daily food intake will look like:

- Lean protein: 2 servings of 4.5–5.5 ounces (see protein list below).

- Fruit: 2 servings per day (see fruit list below).

- Non-starchy vegetables: Unlimited (see non-starchy veggies list below).

- Water: Half your body weight in ounces daily (up to 100 ounces).

- Caffeine: One cup of coffee, black tea, or caffeinated Zevia per day. Most of the Zevia flavors are not caffeinated – check the label carefully.

Protein Options:

- Sirloin steak

- Hamburger (85% lean or better)

- Chicken or turkey (whole or ground, 85% lean or better)

- White fish (tilapia, cod, flounder, sole, haddock)

- Shrimp, scallops, lobster, crab, clams, mussels, oysters)

- Organic tofu

- Veggie burgers (Hilary's is a favorite for its clean ingredients)

- Egg whites (liquid store-bought egg whites are okay)

Fruits:

- Apples (medium)
- Navel oranges
- Berries (1 cup): strawberries, blueberries, raspberries, blackberries
- Lemon (add some to your water – a cup of warm water with lemon in the morning is a great way to start your day)

Non-starchy vegetables: Fresh or Frozen

- Dark green, red, yellow and orange peppers
- Green beans
- Onions
- Mushrooms
- Celery
- Artichoke
- Asparagus
- Celery
- Lettuce
- Kale
- Zucchini
- Yellow Squash
- Tomatoes (technically a fruit, but we think of them as veggies)
- Cucumbers
- Broccoli

- Cauliflower

- Brussel Sprouts

- Carrots

Tips for Week 1:

- Logging Your Weight: Track your daily progress in your Balanced Warrior 30-Day Journal, which you can download from the RESOURCES page at https://30toLife.org or create one yourself. Log weight changes and note anything unusual (like bloating or lack of sleep).

- Logging your weight daily during this Balanced Warrior phase isn't about obsessing over the number; it's about collecting data without drama. It helps you see patterns, trends, and how your body responds to different foods, sleep, stress, or even that extra glass of sparkling water. Daily tracking keeps you connected and honest with yourself, and it helps take the mystery out of what's really going on. And once again, let me remind you, this is not about perfection. It's about awareness. When you approach the scale with curiosity instead of judgment, it becomes a tool for empowerment, not punishment.

- Crowding Out to Crowd In: Fill your plate with non-starchy vegetables to "crowd out" cravings for starchy or fatty foods.

- Stay Positive: If the scale doesn't move one day, that's okay. Weight release is not always linear so keep going!

What to Expect:

In the first few days, you may experience detox symptoms such as headaches, fatigue, or cravings. These are signs that your body is adjusting and healing. By the end of Week 1, most people report increased energy, better sleep, and a reduction in bloating.

Remember: This isn't a quick fix. It's the beginning of a life-changing journey. Stick with it, and you'll see incredible results.

You Are a Warrior — Your Journey Is Real!

Check the Reference page on our website for more information at https://30toLife.org/references.

> ***ProTip***: The first 30 days are all about building a strong foundation. Keep it simple and focus on what foods are helping you rather than what you are temporarily not eating. Stock your kitchen with a variety of Balanced Warrior proteins, fresh vegetables, and flavorful seasonings to keep your meals interesting. Please think of this phase as a gift to your body; you're giving it the reset it deserves. And don't stress about perfection. Progress, not perfection, is the goal. If you stumble, just keep going.

You Are a Warrior — Your Journey Is Real!

My Journey

What small changes can you commit to during this phase? Jot down how you feel about removing certain foods and focusing on hormone balancing. What excites you about starting this Balanced Warrior 30-day balancing?

_____

_____

_____

_____

_____

_____

_____

_____

_____

_____

_____

_____

_____

CHAPTER 22

You Are a Harmony Heroine – Phase Two

"Put some Windex on it." — My Big Fat Greek Wedding

Congratulations! You've completed the full Balanced Warrior phase, and I bet you feel AMAZING. Take a moment to soak it all in: the pride, the accomplishment, and the fact that you gave yourself the gift of health. This is a huge milestone on your journey to a healthier, more vibrant life.

Now, let's address what you may be thinking: you may not have reached your ideal healthy weight yet. That's okay! The Balanced Warrior phase is not designed to be the finish line; it's the foundation. It helped reset your body, balance your stress hormones, and create momentum. The next phase is where you'll continue to release weight while building habits that'll last a lifetime. You have probably guessed it's not as easy as putting some Windex on it. Although spraying foods you would rather not eat, well…maybe not. Let's keep going.

Stepping Into Harmony Heroine Phase – Reintroducing Foods into Your Life

I get it. This next phase might feel scary. That little voice in your head might be whispering, "What if I can't keep this up?" or "What if I lose the progress I've made?" Let me tell you something: if you haven't reached your Ideal Healthy Weight, you will continue to release. If you have reached your IHW, you will maintain it easily and effortlessly.

When I first started reintroducing foods, I was convinced that not only would I stop releasing weight, but I'd also start gaining it back. This fear is so common that I see it over and over with my clients. One client, for example, was so nervous about reintroducing foods after the first 30 days that she outright refused to do it. Her husband, also on the program, had started reintroducing various foods and was progressing. Still, she couldn't shake the fear. It took weeks of coaching, but she finally started adding new foods. She continued to release weight, 48 pounds in total, and she's maintained her ideal weight.

The key is to reintroduce foods systematically, one step at a time. This isn't about rushing to eat all the things you've missed; it's about understanding your body and how it responds to different foods. Pay attention, be patient, and remember this is YOUR journey.

Reintroducing Foods with Confidence

Here are some tips to guide you as you reintroduce foods:

- **Take it slow**: Until you reach your IHW, introduce one new food per week. Once you reach your IHW, you can introduce a new food every three days. Many times, I have made the mistake of jumping right back to eating all the foods I want

152

right away after reducing. It is essential that you slowly reintroduce foods so that you can discover how your body reacts to each food. This gives your body time to adjust and shows how that food affects your weight, mood, digestion, and energy levels. The idea is to reintroduce foods you enjoy eating but haven't been eating for the past 30 days.

- **Keep weighing yourself**: Daily weigh-ins aren't about judgment but awareness. This isn't a diet anymore; it's your lifestyle.

- **Track your observations**: Write in your Balanced Warrior Journal even the smallest changes you notice. Whether it's weight fluctuations, stomach issues, or a surprising burst of energy, these notes are your body's way of communicating with you.

- **Stay hydrated**: Drink half your body weight in ounces of water (up to 100 ounces) daily. As you release weight, your water intake may have adjusted, but hydration remains critical for maintaining balance. I remember how excited I would get when I could reduce my water intake because my weight went down. Silly, I know, but it's the little things that help keep us motivated and focused on our goals.

- **Get moving**: Now that your cortisol is balanced, it's time to embrace movement that makes you feel alive. For me, that's a brisk 2+ mile walk every day. I listen to detective stories while walking; it's my secret motivation! What will yours be? If you were a regular, intense exerciser before the Balanced Warrior phase, you can now go back to running, jogging, lifting, cross-training, or whatever else you were doing prior to the Balanced Warrior phase. Keep an eye on whether you notice the scale going up. You want to stay in balance, so pay attention. You may need to moderate your intense workouts and bring them back slowly.

Gradually reintroducing foods gives your body a chance to communicate what it needs. This isn't just about weight, it's about discovering how certain foods make you feel, both physically and emotionally.

Finding Joy in Movement

Start small if you haven't exercised in a while (or ever). Movement should feel good, not like a chore. Maybe it's dancing in your living room, taking a yoga class, or trying a Barre workout. Start with what you love and build from there.

Remember, movement isn't about punishment; it's about celebrating what your body can do. Movement, like water, is a cornerstone of maintaining your health and releasing weight.

Now that your body is balanced, you're primed to enjoy movement as part of your lifestyle, not as a "have to," but as a "get to." Always check with your healthcare professional before starting a new fitness regimen.

Plateaus – That Dreaded Word

This is the perfect place to talk about the dreaded "plateau." First, let's clarify: a true plateau means the scale hasn't moved in over eight days. Yep, eight days. You've probably noticed a pattern that is uniquely yours during the Balanced Warrior phase. I know I did. I sometimes went a week or more without seeing a release, and then, one to two pounds would drop. Stay the course.

If it's been more than eight days, return to your Balanced Warrior Journal and look. Are you eating the same few foods

154

repeatedly? Variety is key. Are you skipping meals or going too long without eating? Are you moving your body daily, even for 5-10 minutes?

Keep going. You are building a healthy, sustainable lifestyle.

You Are a Warrior — Your Journey Is Real!

Rethinking Your Ideal Healthy Weight

Let's talk about that magic number you have in your head, which you think you need to see on the scale. Most of my clients do this, and I used to as well. But here's the truth: that number is often a mix of fear and self-sabotage. Fear of failure tells us to set a goal that feels "safe," while fear of success whispers that we'll never be able to maintain the weight we truly want.

Here's my advice: let that number go for now. Focus on the bigger picture, your health, how you feel in your body, and your relationship with food. The scale is just one tool; while it can be helpful, it doesn't define your success.

Making Peace with the Scale

I used to think the scale was my worst enemy. How could that little device bring so much misery? But I've learned that the scale isn't the problem. It's a tool, a way to stay accountable and track progress.

Once you reach Phase 3, Freedom Eater, and your IHW, you won't need to weigh yourself daily. Some of my clients continue to weigh themselves every day; that will be a personal choice for you. Two to three times a week is enough to keep you in tune with your body. And if the number fluctuates? That's okay. Fluctuations are part of life. We'll talk more about how to handle them in Chapter 16, but for now, remember: you are in control. The scale is just one piece of the puzzle, and it's here to support you, not define you.

Final Note:

You've already proven to yourself that you can make incredible progress. This next phase is about building on that foundation, one confident step at a time. Trust yourself, trust your body, and trust the process.

> *ProTip*: Transitioning to the next phase after balancing is about trust and curiosity. Reintroduce foods slowly and observe how your body responds. Use your scale as a benchmark. Weigh yourself every day in the Harmony Heroine Phase until you reach your IHW, then two or three times per week. There is no judgment, just experimentation and knowledge.

Movement and water remain your allies; find joyful ways to stay active, whether a daily walk or trying something new. Most importantly, redefine success beyond numbers; focus on your feelings and the sustainable habits you are building. Don't forget to track your non-scale victories.

You Are a Warrior — Your Journey Is Real!

My Journey

How do you feel in your own skin right now? Are you looking to release more excess weight? Go back to your WHY. Has it changed?

_____

_____

_____

_____

_____

_____

_____

_____

_____

_____

_____

_____

_____

_____

CHAPTER 23

Reintroducing Foods – Let's Get Specific

"Everything you see I owe to spaghetti." — Sophia Loren

The Harmony Heroine phase is as much about learning as it is about nourishing. By systematically adding foods back, you'll uncover what works for your body and what might cause inflammation, weight gain, or other unwanted symptoms. This detective work will empower you to craft a personalized, sustainable approach to eating.

When I finished my Balanced Warrior 30-day balancing phase, I wanted to learn more about my body's sensitivities. This curiosity led me to consult a Doctor of Naturopathy for a full allergy and food sensitivity panel. While this isn't necessary for everyone, it opened my eyes to how certain foods uniquely affect me. For instance, I'd avoided lobster for nearly 20 years due to one bad experience where I developed a mild rash after eating it. Turns out, after proper testing,

I wasn't allergic at all! However, I discovered sensitivities to dairy, mussels, beef, and other foods.

Based on this knowledge, I chose to adjust my lifestyle, giving up beef altogether, limiting dairy, and avoiding mussels. This is what worked for me, but your journey will look different. Some of my clients have similar testing done, while others rely on their own experiences to guide them. Either way, reintroducing foods thoughtfully is key to learning what nourishes your body and what might hold you back.

The Importance of Systematic Reintroduction

When you begin adding foods back, you want to do it one step at a time. Jumping back into all your old favorites at once can undo your progress, mask how specific foods affect you, and may lead to weight gain. The process is simple but requires patience and mindfulness.

Think of your scale as a powerful detective tool, it can provide valuable clues about how your body responds to new foods. If you notice the number creeping up after reintroducing a certain food, take note and pause. This doesn't mean you can never eat that food again; it simply gives you insights into how and when to enjoy it (perhaps as part of your Freedom Eater 20%).

Symptoms to Watch For

Food sensitivities or intolerances can manifest in surprising ways. It's not just about weight gain; your body might react with symptoms like:

- Headaches
- Bloating
- Diarrhea or constipation
- Joint pain or achiness

DIETING SUCKS FOR WOMEN OVER 40

- Fatigue or brain fog

Use your 30-Day Balanced Warrior Journal during the Harmony Heroine reintroduction phase to track what you eat, how your body feels, and what the scale tells you. Noticing patterns will help you identify foods that may not serve your long-term goals.

The Basics of Reintroduction

Here's a step-by-step guide for reintroducing foods during the Harmony Heroine phase:

1. **Add One Food at a Time**: Choose one food category or specific food to reintroduce. You may be tempted to add more, but don't let temptation get the best of you. After all, temptation is most likely what got you here in the first place.

2. **Wait Three Days** Before Adding Another Food if you have reached your ideal healthy weight. If not, introduce one new food per week until you reach your IHW. This gives your body time to show any reactions.

3. **Start with Healthy Fats**: These are often the easiest to digest and the most beneficial for overall health. Choose one at a time. Examples:

   - Olive Oil: 1 tablespoon per day (or any other oil)

   - Avocado: Half an avocado per day

   - Almonds: 1 ounce (about 23 almonds) per day

   - Chia Seeds: 1 tablespoon per day

   - Salmon, Tuna or Swordfish (4.5-5.5 ounces per serving)

   - Nut Butters: 2 tablespoons per day (measured, not mounds)

161

- Salad dressing, mayonnaise: 2 tablespoons per day

- Butter: 1 ounce o Note: If a food causes an issue (e.g., almonds lead to weight gain or bloating), note it in your journal and save it for your Freedom Eater 20% indulgences later. REMINDER: The 80/20 Rule is discussed in Chapter 24.

4. **Add Variety to Fruits**: Begin adding more variety of berries (blueberries, raspberries, blackberries) and pears. Melons can follow, but stick to a ½ cup serving. Tropical fruits like mangoes, papayas, and pineapples should be added last, as they contain more sugar.

   - Continue limiting fruit to two servings per day.

5. **Experiment with Dairy (if you consume it)**: Hard cheeses like Parmesan or aged cheddar are a great place to start. Creamier cheeses like Brie or triple cream cheeses should wait for your Freedom Eater 20% because they are higher in fat.

6. **Introduce Healthy Grains Cautiously**: Grains can be tricky since they can trigger weight gain or inflammation. Keep portions small and precise (measure carefully).

   - Examples of 1 serving: (if you have no adverse reaction, you may have two servings per day)
     o Quinoa: ½ cup cooked
     o Oats: ½ cup cooked
     o Brown Rice: ⅓ cup cooked
     o Buckwheat: ½ cup cooked

7. **Add Starchy Vegetables**: Now it's time to add back some favorites. Like with all foods you are reintroducing, always

DIETING SUCKS FOR WOMEN OVER 40

leave 3 days between foods the first time you reintroduce them. Corn, peas, and beans (⅓ cup cooked) and squashes like acorn or butternut (½ cup cooked). Potatoes (white, red, or sweet) should also be limited to ½ cup cooked and one serving per day. Many people find that white potato causes inflammation. Pay close attention to any joint pain when reintroducing white potatoes.

8. **Breads**: Whole-grain breads are best. Look for at least 3 grams of fiber and no more than 3 grams of added sugar. I like Dave's 60-calorie 21 Whole Grains & Seeds. Experiment and note any adverse sensations.

9. **Sugar**: If you have reached your IHW, you can experiment with adding back a minimum amount of sugar. This would include a tablespoon of honey, maple syrup, or brown sugar.

If sugar is an emotional trigger for you, skip this. You can have your sugar as part of the Freedom Eater 20%.

Your Detective Work

This phase is all about discovering how specific foods affect you. For example, one of my clients tried almonds and noticed her weight spiked the next day. She double-checked the ingredients and discovered no added oils or salt, and tried again three days later, with the same result. Almonds, she learned, were not a good fit for her, so she decided to only indulge in them occasionally as a Freedom Eater. I have recently realized that almonds and almond milk make me gassy and bloated. I have decided to eliminate them from my diet. Cashews?? – that's another story and those are for my 20%. More on this in our next Chapter.

Use this time to learn how your body responds to different foods, and don't be discouraged if something you love doesn't "work" for now. You are in control and can always choose how to enjoy it later.

Taste Bud Transformation

Have you noticed how your taste buds have changed during the Balanced Warrior 30-day balancing? Many clients report that foods like berries, which seemed "okay" before, now taste incredibly sweet. This is a sign that your body has detoxed from processed sugars and is now appreciating the natural flavors of whole foods. Celebrate this shift, it's a sign of progress!

A New Relationship with Food

Reintroducing foods isn't just about identifying sensitivities; it's about building a new relationship with food. You'll start to notice which foods nourish your body, give you energy, and make you feel great. You'll also see which foods leave you feeling sluggish, bloated, or unsatisfied.

Remember, this process is personal. Your goal is to create a lifestyle that allows you to feel strong, vibrant, and in control. Trust the process and take your time.

This is a critical step toward becoming a Freedom Eater and living life diet-free. Please take it slow. Use your self-hypnosis daily to reinforce all your new habits, confidence, and healthy lifestyle. Review Chapter 9, Fear of Failure and Fear of Success, and Chapter 2, Emotional Triggers to reinforce your commitment.

Read your WHY daily and rework it, if needed.

You Are a Warrior — Your Journey Is Real!

ProTip: Reintroducing foods is your opportunity to learn what truly nourishes your body. Take it slow, introduce one food at a time, and use your 30-Day Balanced Warrior Journal to document how each addition makes you feel physically and mentally. I kept a handwritten log for a year as I added foods to my diet. I also had testing done to see what foods I was physically sensitive to. Pay attention to symptoms like bloating, fatigue, or cravings to spot sensitivities. Remember, this isn't about perfection but about building a sustainable, personalized approach to eating. Balance and patience lead to lasting success.

My Journey

What foods are you most interested in reintroducing? Start listing foods to be reintroduced over the next four weeks.

_____

_____

_____

_____

_____

_____

_____

_____

_____

_____

_____

_____

_____

CHAPTER 24

Freedom Eater — 80/20 Way of Life — Phase Three

"If life gives you limes, make margaritas."
— Jimmy Buffet

Once you've reached your Ideal Healthy Weight (IHW), it's time to shift into the Freedom Eater 80/20 way of life. It does not matter how long it takes you to achieve your Ideal Healthy Weight. I have worked with clients who wanted to release 8-10 pounds and those whose goal was over 100 pounds. This is YOUR JOURNEY. Once you reach your goal weight, it's time to focus on maintaining it in an effortless, sustainable, and enjoyable way. This is where the Freedom Eater 80/20 lifestyle and the concept of a cushion come into play.

The 80/20 Lifestyle

The Freedom Eater 80/20 lifestyle is about creating balance: 80% of the time, you stick with the healthy habits and foods that support your weight and well-being. The other 20% is for indulging in the foods and experiences you love, guilt-free.

This isn't about being perfect or restrictive, it's about enjoying life while keeping your body balanced. Whether it's a piece of pizza, a cocktail with friends, or dessert on a special occasion, the Freedom Eater 20% gives you the freedom to indulge while staying in control.

Here are some examples of living as a Freedom Eater.

1. The Birthday Cake Rule

Susan spent most of her adult life skipping cake at parties. "I'm good," she'd say, while silently dying for a slice of chocolate cake with buttercream frosting.

Now? Susan eats the cake, if she really wants it.

She doesn't eat cake every night. She doesn't use it as a reward or a coping mechanism. But when her best friend turned 60 and they brought out that bakery-fresh triple chocolate masterpiece, she said yes. She enjoyed every bite, no guilt, no second-guessing.

That's the Freedom Eater 80/20: saying yes to something special, knowing it won't throw you off track, it is the track.

2. The Tuesday Night Pivot

Karen planned to make grilled salmon and broccoli for dinner. But her kid had a meltdown, her dog ran out the front door, and by 7:30, she only had energy for picking up a rotisserie chicken and a bagged salad from the store. While chicken is a great choice for your 80%, store-bought rotisserie chicken is part of your 20%. Some stores add ingredients to rotisserie chicken, such as sugar or honey, etc. that you don't want in your 80%.

Did she blow it? Nope. That was her Freedom Eater 20%.

She didn't hit the burger and fries drive-thru. She didn't order pizza and eat the whole thing. She made the best choice she could in the moment, without spiraling.

Freedom Eater 80/20 means flexibility. It represents progress, not perfection.

3. The Ice Cream Test

Lauren keeps a pint of mint chip in her freezer. A year ago, she wouldn't have dared. She'd have eaten the whole thing in one sitting, then bought another and "started over Monday."

Now? It takes her two weeks to finish it. Sometimes she has a few bites. Sometimes none. It's not forbidden anymore. It's just… ice cream.

When food loses its power, you get yours back.

That's Freedom Eater 80/20. That's freedom.

4. The All-You-Can-Eat Buffet Test

Diane used to dread all-inclusive vacations. Not because she didn't love the beach, but because of the food. Buffets, bottomless drinks, dessert tables that seemed to whisper, "Go ahead, you're on vacation…"

She'd start strong with fruit and eggs at breakfast… but by day three, it was pancakes, piña coladas before noon, and that creeping feeling of "I've blown it, so what's one more croissant?"

But this time was different.

Diane still enjoyed herself. She had the cocktail. She tried the dessert. But she also walked the beach every morning, drank plenty of water, and chose foods that made her feel good 80% of the time, without restriction, guilt, or that old familiar spiral.

She came home feeling refreshed, not regretful.

Because Freedom Eater 80/20 isn't about rules, it's about freedom with intention.

5. The Chips & Salsa Standoff

Jill knew the chips basket was trouble the moment it hit the table. She was out with friends at her favorite Mexican place where the margaritas are the size of a toddler's head and the salsa is worth writing poetry about.

Old Jill would've gone all in with two baskets of chips, a frozen mango margarita, enchiladas smothered in cheese, and a side of shame.

But Freedom Eater Jill? She took a breath. She enjoyed a handful of chips, slowly. Sipped her margarita without rushing to reorder. And when dinner came, she swapped the rice for extra grilled veggies, not because she "had to," but because she wanted to feel good the next day.

She left satisfied, not stuffed. Happy, not guilty. Powerful, not punished.

Freedom Eater 80/20 doesn't mean no chips. It means you decide how the night ends, and it's not with regret.

I can relate to all these stories. They are real-life examples of what living a life diet-free can look like. For me, 20% is often a bagel from my favorite local bagel place. Or maybe dinner out with my husband at a local restaurant. Most of my 20% is done when we travel. Whether it's a day trip to New York City or a week of all-inclusiveness, it's usually when I am away from home. You will have your own experiences, and I'd love for you to share them with me at Debbie@30toLife.org.

The Cushion

Let's be real: life happens. You're going to have vacations, celebrations, weddings, birthdays, and holidays. You may even have weeks where you eat more out of convenience or indulgence than balance. That's okay. With the Freedom Eater 80/20 lifestyle, your body will naturally regulate itself if you have a strategy.

One way to make this lifestyle even more stress-free is to build in a 2–4-pound cushion once you reach your Ideal Healthy Weight. This gives you a little wiggle room to fluctuate without panicking or feeling like you've "failed."

How the Cushion Works

When you've been living your Freedom Eater 80/20 lifestyle and maintaining your ideal healthy weight, you'll notice that even after vacations or indulgent weekends, your weight may go up only slightly, and it comes back down quickly once you return to your usual 80%.

For example, I recently took an all-inclusive vacation where I ate and drank more than I normally would. When I got home, I knew the scale would be up. I waited two days before weighing myself, knowing that some of the initial gain was simply water retention from the extra alcohol, salt, sugar, and fat. When I finally stepped on the scale, I was only two pounds up, which released in just a few days.

The key here is knowing yourself. Waiting two days helps me avoid falling into a self-sabotaging spiral. If I see the scale go up too much right after vacation, my saboteur might chime in with, "See, nothing works, you've gained weight again. Might as well keep eating."

But by waiting and sticking to my Freedom Eater 80% for a few days, I can confidently say, "See, a vacation and only two pounds up. I am a Warrior and My Journey is Real."

Knowing Your Psychology

Everyone's approach to the scale is different, and knowing what works best for you is crucial. Some feel motivated by weighing themselves the morning after vacation, no matter the number. Others, like me, benefit from waiting a couple of days to see the more accurate picture.

Either way, immediately returning to your Freedom Eater 80% lifestyle is the most critical thing.

Why Your Weight May Fluctuate

After an indulgent vacation or weekend, the scale might show a gain of 3–5 pounds (or more). Here's why:

- **Salt**: Higher salt intake leads to water retention, making you feel bloated and heavier.

- **Sugar and Fat**: Extra sugar and fat can cause temporary inflammation and bloating.

- **Alcohol**: Most of us who do drink alcohol indulge more on the weekends and on vacation.

The good news is that once you're back to your usual eating and hydration habits, your body will naturally release the excess water and inflammation.

The Role of Movement and Water

Even during indulgent periods, keeping up with some movement and staying hydrated can make a big difference. For example, your body will stay more balanced if you're walking on the beach during vacation or hiking while sightseeing. Drinking plenty of water, half your body weight in ounces (up to 100 ounces), will help flush out toxins and reduce bloating. We always travel with water in the car and ask for a case when we go to our all-inclusive vacation spot.

Practical Tips for Maintaining Your Cushion

Here's how to make the most of your Freedom Eater 80/20 lifestyle while keeping your cushion intact:

1. **Plan Your Indulgences**: Save your 20% for special occasions or treats that truly bring you joy. For example, enjoy that glass of wine with dinner, a decadent dessert, or a slice of pizza, but be mindful of when and how often you indulge.

2. **Stay Active**: Find ways to move your body even during vacations or holidays. Whether walking, dancing, or yoga, movement helps balance your energy and body.

3. **Listen to Your Body**: Pay attention to how you feel after indulgent periods. Do you notice bloating, are your rings tight, or fatigue? Use those signals as gentle reminders to return to your 80%.

4. **Weigh Yourself Strategically**: Decide whether weighing yourself right after vacation motivates you or if waiting two days feels better for your mindset. There's no right or wrong answer; it's just what works for you. Tip: Do not wait more than four days to weigh yourself. Do not even think that you can judge "by my clothes." To live diet-free, you must face your friendly scale.

5. **Get Back to Your 80% Right Away**: After indulgent periods, return to your usual eating habits the next day. Focus on non-starchy vegetables, lean proteins, and plenty of water.

Craving Your 80%

I hear something from clients all the time: "After a few days of indulgence, I start craving my usual healthy meals."

Your body thrives on balance. When you've been eating indulgent foods for a few days, you might notice that your rings feel tight, your skin looks a little off, or your sleep isn't as restful. These subtle signals are your body's way of encouraging you to return to the foods and habits that make you feel good.

After a week of eating out, I start craving the simple turkey burger my husband makes every week. It's a reminder that your body knows what it needs; you just have to listen.

Final Thoughts

The Freedom Eater 80/20 lifestyle and the idea of a cushion are all about freedom, flexibility, and sustainability. By giving yourself room to enjoy life's pleasures while staying mindful of balance, you'll easily maintain your Ideal Healthy Weight.

So, enjoy yourself the next time you're on vacation or celebrating a special occasion. Relish the food, savor the drinks, and know your body can bounce back.

This isn't a "diet" anymore; it's your new way of life.

You Are a Warrior — Your Journey Is Real!

ProTip: The Freedom Eater, 80/20 lifestyle is your ticket to balance and sustainability. Focus on sticking with healthy habits 80% of the time and enjoy indulgences guilt-free during the other 20%. Use the concept of a "cushion," a 2–4-pound range above your Ideal Healthy Weight, as a safety net that allows for natural fluctuations. If you still see your overweight person staring back from your mirror, WORK ON YOUR SUBCONSCIOUS. You will maintain your Ideal Healthy Weight easily and effortlessly.

YOU ARE A WARRIOR

YOUR JOURNEY IS REAL!

YOU DID IT!

My Journey

Reflect on three things you have learned about yourself on this journey to your ideal healthy weight. How has your attitude toward food changed? What would you tell your young self about dieting?

_____

_____

_____

_____

_____

_____

_____

_____

_____

_____

_____

_____

_____

PART 6

ONGOING SUPPORT TOOLS

CHAPTER 25
Self-Hypnosis Steps 1-3

"It is the brain, the little grey cells on which one must rely. One must seek the truth within—not without."
— Agatha Christie, *The Mysterious Affair at Styles*

Self-hypnosis is a remarkable technique for relaxation, boosting confidence, improving sleep, and embedding powerful, positive suggestions into your subconscious mind. Here, I'll guide you through the three steps of self-hypnosis as they were taught to me during my training. This transformative process unfolds over three weeks, and each step builds upon the last.

A Brief Introduction to Hypnosis

Before diving into the steps, let's take a moment to understand the modality of hypnosis. Hypnosis has long been misrepresented in popular culture. For example, if you're a fan of Sherlock Holmes, you might recall the 1945 film The Woman in Green, in which hypnosis is dubiously portrayed as a tool for committing murder. While entertaining, such depictions are far from accurate.

Modern science tells us that hypnosis cannot make you do anything you wouldn't willingly do out of hypnosis. This understanding dates to Franz Anton Mesmer, an Austrian physician whose theories of "animal magnetism" laid the groundwork for what we now know as hypnosis. Mesmer lived from 1734 to 1815, and his legacy even gave us the word "mesmerize."

Many people associate hypnosis with stage shows where participants perform silly antics. While these shows are real, stage hypnotists are highly skilled in identifying eager and willing individuals to participate. I volunteered to be a subject at a hypnosis annual conference. There were 12 of us on the stage. Only 3 of us were great subjects and performed the silly tasks that the hypnotist suggested. It's essential to note that in a therapeutic setting, hypnosis is a tool for self-improvement, not entertainment. It is equally important to know that most people can benefit from hypnosis. You do not have to get into a very deep state (as my three colleagues on stage did) to benefit tremendously from hypnosis. In hypnosis, you are always aware and in control.

Have you ever driven to a destination, only to realize you don't remember the journey? That's a form of hypnosis called "highway hypnosis." Your mind was relaxed, but you would have instantly reacted to any danger. Similarly, during self-hypnosis, your conscious mind takes a break, allowing your subconscious to absorb positive suggestions.

Step 1: Pre-Sleep Technique (Days 1-14)

Begin your self-hypnosis journey by establishing a simple pre-sleep routine:

1. When you are in bed, just before falling asleep, repeat the following suggestion ten times: "Every day, in every way, I am better and better."

2. Avoid falling asleep mid-way through the repetitions. A helpful trick is to press down with each finger of your right hand for the first five repetitions, then with each finger of your left hand for the next five. This tactile action helps keep you focused.

This step lays the foundation for programming yourself with positive suggestions. Stick with it for seven days, and you'll likely notice positive changes in your mindset and energy levels.

Step 2: Daily Hypnotic Relaxation (Days 8-14)

Continue with your pre-sleep routine while adding two daily self-hypnosis sessions. These sessions should last 3-5 minutes each and can be done in the morning, midday, or early evening. Continue with Step 1 while you are doing Step 2.

1. **Find a Comfortable Spot**: To ground yourself, sit in a chair with your back supported and your feet flat on the floor.

2. **Focus Your Gaze**: Pick a spot opposite you, slightly above eye level.

3. **Breathe Deeply**: Take three deep breaths. On the third breath, hold it for three seconds as you count backwards: 3...2...1.

4. **Relax**: Close your eyes, exhale, and allow yourself to drift into a deep, relaxed state.

5. **Count Backwards**: Visualize or imagine writing each number on a blackboard or whiteboard as you count slowly from 25 down to 1.

To exit hypnosis, simply count forward from 1 to 3, bringing yourself back to full awareness. This practice reinforces relaxation and prepares your mind to accept positive suggestions.

Step 3: Embedding Positive Suggestions (Days 15+)

After two weeks of practice, you're ready to integrate positive suggestions into your routine. You may now discontinue Step 2. Many clients continue Step I as they enjoy this positive affirmation during pre-sleep. Here's how to make the most of this step:

1. Use an Index Card: Write your suggestion on a 3x5 index card. Avoid digital alternatives; the tactile act of writing reinforces your intent. Also, you do not want to be "dropping" your cell phone. Keep a card in your purse, car, or anywhere easily accessible.

2. Craft Your Suggestion (see examples below): Ensure your suggestion is:

   - Positive: Focus on what you want to achieve.

   - Believable: Choose a suggestion you can genuinely accept. o Simple: Keep it clear and concise and in the present tense.

   - Measurable: Include a way to track progress.

   - Rewarding: Attach a small reward to your progress.

Examples of powerful suggestions include:

- "I enjoy making healthy food choices daily and feel proud of my commitment to nourishing my body."

- "I feel lighter and more energetic with every step I take, and I love how my clothes fit me comfortably."

- "I am strong and in control of my eating habits and celebrate my progress with each healthy meal I eat."

Rewards can be as simple as treating yourself to a manicure, buying a new blouse, or purchasing a kitchen gadget that supports your healthy lifestyle. They can also be completely free, like taking a quiet walk in nature or giving yourself permission to enjoy a guilt-free afternoon nap. Celebrating small victories keeps you motivated and reinforces the positive changes you've made.

1. Sit down and choose a spot opposite you, slightly above eye level. Hold your index card in front of the spot and read the suggestion to yourself 3 times. Make sure the words on the card are believable to you and allow yourself to imagine accomplishing what is written on the card. Use your imagination.

2. Now, drop the card and take a deep breath. Exhale. Hold your second deep breath and count backward from 3 to 1. Close your eyes, exhale, and enter deep hypnosis.

3. Instead of counting backward from 25 to 1, allow the suggestion to repeat over and over in your subconscious mind. At the same time, imagine, pretend, or visualize that you are carrying out your suggestion. At times, the words start to break up and become fragmented. This is normal; you still impart these words deep into your subconscious.

You've now equipped yourself with the tools to embrace self-hypnosis. Make it a daily habit, and you'll uncover a relaxed, empowered version of yourself capable of achieving your goals with confidence and ease.

ProTip: Self-hypnosis is like planting seeds in a garden; you set the foundation for growth with every session. Start small and be consistent, even if it's just two minutes a day. Use tactile triggers to stay focused, like pressing your fingers during repetitions. Keep your suggestions in the present, positive, simple, and achievable. For example: "I feel lighter and stronger with each step I take." Write them down, yes, an old-school index card works best! Remember, this is your time to nurture your mindset and create a positive shift.

You Are a Warrior — Your Journey Is Real!

My Journey

What thoughts or beliefs have been holding you back? Reflect on how you can use the power of your 'little grey cells' to rewrite those thoughts and steer yourself toward success.

_____

_____

_____

_____

_____

_____

_____

_____

_____

_____

_____

_____

_____

_____

_____

CHAPTER 26

Sleep: Your Secret Weapon

"I'm just a guy who loves to sleep. Sleeping is the best recovery that you can possibly have. It's better than any other recovery you can do." — LeBron James

---

I am always skeptical when people say, "I only need three hours of sleep a night." While I believe they can function that way, I wonder: Is that a healthy or sustainable way to live? Do you really need 20 hours a day to work? To me, it sounds like they're sacrificing something critical, the rejuvenating, healing power of sleep. It's almost like bragging about not taking a vacation in five years. Hmmm... If you're one of those who prides themselves on burning the candle at both ends, listen up: Sleep (and downtime from work) is essential for a healthy lifestyle.

I chose to include a quote from LeBron James at the start of this chapter because, a few years ago, I listened to his three-part audio on the Calm App. I'm fascinated by LeBron's skills on the court, approach to recovery, and philanthropy. He's serious about getting lots of sleep daily because he understands that sleep is as vital to his performance as practice or nutrition. If one of the greatest athletes of all time prioritizes sleep, shouldn't we?

How Much Sleep Are You Getting?

So, let's talk about you. How much sleep are you really getting each night?

If you own an Apple Watch, Samsung Watch, Fitbit, or other fitness tracker, it might be monitoring your sleep patterns. I stopped charging my Apple Watch at night to see how much sleep I was getting. While the accuracy of these devices can be debated, they offer valuable insights into your habits.

If you're unsure how much sleep you get, consider tracking it for a week. You might be surprised that you're averaging far less than you thought. And that lack of sleep could be holding you back, not just in your weight-release journey but in every aspect of your health and well-being.

The Sleep-Weight Connection

Sleep affects weight loss; it's not just about feeling tired the next day. According to a Harvard Medical School Health blog, people who sleep less actually consume more calories. Lack of sleep messes with the hormones that regulate appetite and fullness.

You can find the blog on the References page here https://30toLife. org/references.

Think about it: Have you ever eaten something sugary or carb-heavy to stay awake when you were exhausted? I have. It's almost like your body screams, "Give me energy now!" And the quickest fix often comes in the form of sweets or junk food. The problem is, it's a vicious cycle. Those unhealthy choices spike your blood sugar, give you a quick burst of energy, and leave you feeling even more tired later.

For some people, exhaustion does the opposite. Instead of reaching for food, they skip meals altogether, which slows down metabolism and further drains energy. I am not one of those people who can be exhausted and just go to bed. I don't ever go to bed hungry which can lead to food right before bed. I make a concerted effort not to let that happen. It's something you want to pay attention to. When we are tired, we also don't feel like moving our bodies.

That's a double whammy when it comes to weight management.

Why We Don't Sleep Enough

If it's common sense that sleep is essential, why aren't most of us getting enough?

For women, perimenopause and menopause are often to blame. Sleep challenges during these phases are widespread, and night sweats don't exactly make for peaceful slumber. The good news? Hormonal balancing, like what you do in the Balanced Warrior 30-Day Balancing Program, can dramatically reduce or even eliminate night sweats over time. But for now, let's look at the other factors that may interfere with your sleep.

Common Sleep Disruptors

Do any of these sound familiar?

- **Stress and overthinking**: Lying awake at night, replaying work scenarios, or worrying about the next day.

- **Late caffeine**: That afternoon coffee or tea that seemed like a good idea at 3 p.m. might haunt you at bedtime.

- **Late-night eating**: Eating a heavy meal within two hours of bedtime can disrupt digestion and make it harder to fall asleep.

- **Waiting up for kids or loved ones**: Whether it's a teenager out with friends or a partner working late, waiting up for someone can wreak havoc on your sleep schedule.

- **Room temperature**: Did you know the optimal sleeping temperature is 65 degrees Fahrenheit / 18.33 degrees Celsius? According to the Sleep Foundation, if your room is too warm, it could be keeping you awake. You can find the blog on the RESOURCES page here https://30toLife.org/references.

- **Electronics**: Scrolling through your phone or watching TV in bed can stimulate your brain and interfere with melatonin production.

- **Alcohol**: While a glass of wine might make you feel relaxed, too much alcohol can disrupt your sleep cycles, leaving you feeling groggy the next day.

How to Sleep Better

The good news is that you can improve sleep with little effort and consistency. Here are some practical tips to help you get the rest your body craves:

1. **Stick to a schedule**: Commit to going to bed and waking up at the same time every day, even on weekends. This consistency helps regulate your internal clock.

2. **Create a bedtime ritual**: Read, meditate, take a warm bath, or practice self-hypnosis before bed. Find what relaxes you and make it part of your nightly routine.

3. **Limit screen time**: Put your phone down at least 30 minutes before bed. And if you have a TV in your bedroom, skip the news or anything too stimulating.

4. **Cool your room**: Aim for a cooler sleeping environment, around 65-68 degrees Fahrenheit. Use a fan if necessary or invest in cooling bedding. Now we can have beds that regulate temperature. I don't have one and my husband and I are very different. He is sleeping in sweatpants, sweatshirt, and two blankets. I am sleeping in a t-shirt and have a fan near me.

5. **Watch your diet**: Avoid heavy meals, alcohol, or caffeine before bedtime. Instead, opt for light, sleep-promoting snacks like a banana or a handful of almonds.

6. **Move during the day**: Regular movement, whether walking, yoga, or another activity, can help you sleep better at night. Just avoid intense exercise right before bed.

7. **Address pain or discomfort**: If aches and pains are keeping you awake, speak with your healthcare provider. Pain relief is essential for quality sleep.

8. **Experiment with naps**: Some people can nap during the day without affecting their nighttime sleep. If you're not one of them, skip the naps and focus on a whole night's rest. I am not a napper. If I do nap, I cannot sleep that night, so it doesn't work for me. I have known people who can grab a 10-minute catnap anywhere and wake up totally refreshed.

I have always been envious of them.

Sleep and Your Weight-Release Journey

One of the first things clients tell me during the Balanced Warrior 30-Day balancing phase is how much better they're sleeping. They wake up refreshed, energized, and ready to take on the day. It's no coincidence. Your body naturally craves rest as you balance your hormones, reduce inflammation, and release excess weight.

Remember, this whole journey is about you. Sleep is a gift you're giving yourself, a chance for your body to heal, recharge, and thrive. So, experiment with these tips, find what works for you, and enjoy the many benefits of a great night's sleep.

> *ProTip*: Sleep is essential for recharging your body and mind, but making your bedroom a sanctuary doesn't have to mean ditching all electronics. If your phone is your go-to for calming music or meditation apps, set it to "Do Not Disturb" or "Sleep" mode and keep it away from your pillow to minimize disruptions. I have one YouTube account that I upgraded so I can listen to a sleep meditation, and it will play all night without ads cutting in. Likewise, a TV is fine as long as you're watching something relaxing, NEVER the news or anything scary or violent. The key is to create a calming environment that helps you unwind. Remember, even minor adjustments to your sleep routine can make a big difference in your overall well-being.

You Are a Warrior — Your Journey Is Real!

My Journey

How does your sleep affect your mood, energy, and eating patterns?
Write one or two changes you will make today to improve your sleep
habits.

_____

_____

_____

_____

_____

_____

_____

_____

_____

_____

_____

_____

_____

_____

_____

_____

CHAPTER 27

My Vitamin Ritual

"Look! A peanut. Come on, eat it. It's got lots of
vitamins. It'll give you a lot of... pep."
— Timothy Q. Mouse, *Dumbo*

Do you take vitamins and supplements? I've switched between them over the years, but since beginning my weight release journey, I've stayed consistent. Supplements have been a helpful addition to my routine, but I want to remind you that this is your journey, and what works for me may not work for you.

I am not a nutritionist, dietitian, or medical practitioner, so please consult a qualified healthcare provider to determine what supplements (if any) are right for you. I worked with a naturopathic doctor, and blood work revealed specific deficiencies and sensitivities in my body. This helped me choose vitamins and supplements tailored to my needs, and I recommend you do the same.

The World of Supplements

You've probably noticed the constant buzz around new supplements claiming to melt fat, curb cravings, or boost your metabolism. It's overwhelming, and let's be honest, some of us have tried more than a few! Here's a short list of popular supplements often linked to weight loss:

- Green Tea Extract – Thought to boost metabolism and fat burning.

- Garcinia Cambogia – Said to reduce fat storage and control appetite.

- Omega-3 Fatty Acids (Fish Oil) – Helps reduce inflammation and can support belly fat loss when paired with exercise.

- Vitamin D – Linked to hormone balance and better fat regulation, particularly for those with a deficiency.

- Berberine – Known for improving insulin sensitivity, reducing fat storage, and balancing blood sugar.

- Probiotics – A healthy gut can support better weight management and reduce bloating.

- Apple Cider Vinegar (ACV) – May suppress appetite and reduce body fat.

This is by no means an endorsement of any supplement on this list, but it reflects what's currently popular in the health and wellness world. Now, let me share what works for me. My Daily Vitamin Routine

Here's what I take every day:

- Vitamin D

- Methylated B Vitamins (for better absorption—my blood tests showed I don't absorb B vitamins well).

- Omega-3 Fatty Acids

- Probiotic

- Berberine

- And of course, caffeine (yes, caffeine is a supplement) from my daily coffee (but in moderation!).

These have become my staples, but they may not be right for you. Everyone's body is unique, and that's why getting professional advice is so important.

Choosing the Right Supplements

Once you know which supplements are best for you, you must be selective about what brands you buy. Not all supplements are created equal! Here's what I look for when choosing vitamins and supplements:

1. **Third-Party Testing**: Look for certifications from NSF International, USP (U.S. Pharmacopeia), or ConsumerLab. These organizations independently test products for purity, potency, and safety.

2. **Ingredient Transparency**: The label should clearly list all ingredients, including the source (natural vs. synthetic) and any fillers or binders. Avoid anything with artificial additives, colors, or sweeteners.

3. **Bioavailability**: Choose forms that your body can absorb easily.

For example:

- Vitamin D3 is more easily absorbed than D2.

- Methylated B vitamins are ideal if you have absorption issues.

4. **Dosage and Potency**: Ensure the dosage aligns with your needs and doesn't exceed safe limits. More isn't always better; excessive intake can be harmful.

5. **Reputable Brands**: Stick with brands with a strong reputation for quality and transparency. Research reviews and ask your healthcare provider for recommendations.

6. **Country of Origin**: Supplements made in the USA, Canada, or EU countries often adhere to stricter regulations. Look for "Made in a GMP-certified facility" on the label.

7. **Allergen Information**: Check for allergens like gluten, soy, dairy, or shellfish if you have sensitivities.

8. **Expiration Date**: Ensure your supplements are fresh and effective throughout your intended use.

Be Wary of Low-Cost Options

I understand that budget matters, but cheap supplements may contain fillers or not provide the necessary potency. Balance quality with affordability. Remember, this is your health we're talking about.

For more detailed advice, visit trusted resources like the National Center for Complementary and Integrative Health (NCCIH). You can find the information on the References page on our website https://30toLife.org/references.

A Note on Experimentation

Supplements like homeopathic drops can be intriguing, especially if they claim to help with appetite or cravings. I've experimented with them myself, but let me be clear: they're not magic. They work best with a balanced food plan, regular movement, and a positive mindset. Always check with a healthcare professional to be sure you are utilizing the best supplements for you.

Personalize Your Plan

Here's the most crucial part of this discussion: you are unique. Your supplements should support your body's needs, whether boosting energy, balancing hormones, or addressing deficiencies. Keep track with your 30-Day Balanced Warrior journal of what you take and how it affects you. This will help you fine-tune your routine as you progress on your journey.

You Are a Warrior — Your Journey Is Real!

ProTip: Supplements can be a powerful addition to your wellness routine but are not one-size-fits-all. Always prioritize quality over quantity, and choose third-party tested brands with clear, transparent ingredients. Consult a healthcare professional to identify your body's needs and avoid jumping on every trend. Supplements are not magic; it may take months to see actual benefits. Pay attention to how you feel and give supplements time to work for you. Remember: they're just one piece of the puzzle in your journey to health.

You Are a Warrior — Your Journey Is Real!

My Journey

What supplements or vitamins are you currently taking, and how do they support your health? Reflect on what you might add or change.

_____

_____

_____

_____

_____

_____

_____

_____

_____

_____

_____

_____

_____

PART 7

SUPPORTING MATERIAL

CHAPTER 28

For the Boys

"The only place success comes before work is in the dictionary." — Vince Lombardi

"I guess, to tell you the truth, I've never had much of a desire to grow facial hair. I think I've managed to play quarterback just fine without a mustache."
— Peyton Manning

I wanted to include a chapter specifically for men because, while this book is primarily written for women, men have been incredibly successful with my program. Why the football quotes? Why not?

Women are often the catalyst for inspiring the men in their lives to pursue better health. If you have a man who can stand to release some excess weight, leave this chapter lying around. Or, better yet, partner with him so you both get healthier together.

I've also noticed that men have taken more personal responsibility for their health in recent years. This is excellent news, as men often see faster, more dramatic results once they commit to a program. However, there are also a few key differences between men and women regarding weight release that are worth addressing.

Why Weight Loss Is Marketed Primarily to Women

It's no secret that women are the driving force behind the massive weight loss industry. According to a March 2024 blog on Market-Research.com, "The total U.S. weight loss market is estimated to have grown to an historic peak of $90 billion in 2023, boosted by GLP-1 weight loss drugs." The link to this blog can be found on the RESOURCES page at https://30toLife.org/resources.

Women tend to purchase more weight loss products than men, so it's no surprise that most marketing targets women. Whether this is a case of "chicken or the egg," women responding to marketing, or companies responding to demand, it's clear that social pressures to "look young and thin" play a significant role. These pressures fuel the search for the magic "diet elixir."

Men, on the other hand, often come to me for different reasons:

- Their doctor has told them they need to lose weight.
- They're feeling tired and want more energy.
- They've seen a woman in their life succeed with my program and want to give it a try for themselves.

Whatever the reason, if you're a man reading this, congratulations! You've already taken the first step toward improving your health. Men benefit faster and more dramatically from my Balanced Warrior 30-day balancing program.

Why Men Lose Weight Faster Than Women

It's not just a myth; men really do release weight faster than women. Here's why:

- **Muscle Mass**: Men naturally have lean muscle mass, increasing their resting metabolic rate and allowing them to burn more calories, even at rest.

- **Testosterone**: This hormone plays a significant role in building and maintaining muscle, contributing to calorie burn.

- **Compartmentalization**: As Brentwood MD explains in their article, "Is It Easier for Men to Lose Weight?":

"Men's ability to compartmentalize allows them to focus on weight loss tasks separately from emotional or social pressures around body image, a difference that can influence adherence and success rates in weight loss programs."

A link to this article can be found on the RESOURCES at https://30toLife.org/resources.

That's not to say that men don't face challenges with food or emotional eating; they do. However, they often seem more capable of "pushing it aside" once they've decided to release weight and get healthier.

The Competitive Edge

Many men I've worked with bring a competitive mindset to weight release. Whether it's being competitive with themselves or with others, this mindset often drives them to stick to the program and see quick results.

For example:

- Mark came to me wanting to lose weight and lower his cholesterol. His cholesterol dropped 53 points in just three weeks, an unusual but fantastic result that shocked and thrilled his doctor. He was able to go off his cholesterol medication and has kept the weight off for over two years.

- Another male client, who owned a fitness center, came to us because he wanted to cut sugar from his diet. He called himself a "sugaraholic" and knew he needed help. His 30 day balancing program helped him stop eating sugar and lose 19.5 pounds, even though he initially didn't think he needed to release much weight.

A man's ability to compartmentalize and focus on their goals often makes them highly successful in my program. They tend to stick with the plan faithfully, releasing weight more quickly and consistently than women.

A Difference in Priorities

Physiologically, men's bodies work differently from women's. Testosterone, lean muscle mass, and a higher resting metabolic rate contribute to faster weight release.

But during my years working with women and men, I've concluded that there's more to it. Men often approach weight loss with a different set of priorities. While women are often motivated by societal pressures to "look a certain way," men seem more driven by:

- A desire to improve their health (e.g., coming off medications).

- A competitive urge to meet goals or "win" at weight loss.
- Practical motivations include having more energy or feeling better overall.

Historically, many men (especially over 40) weren't as focused on their appearance, instead prioritizing careers, making money, or achieving power. While this has shifted in recent years, with younger men paying more attention to their appearance, it's still common for men to approach weight release with a more results-driven mindset.

It is encouraging that over the past few years, I have spoken to more and more men who are just as motivated as women to be healthy and slender and look and feel younger. I don't know if this is a new trend for men or if they are more open to speaking about their weight and health.

Couples and Weight Loss

When couples do my program together, I often see a playful competitiveness that keeps them motivated. One couple I worked with tied almost weekly during their weight release journey. They enjoyed the process together and supported each other, which made it easier to stick to the plan.

I highly recommend that couples go through the program together. It's a great way to provide mutual support and simplify meal planning. My husband joined me to support my efforts, and in the process, he released 53 pounds and came off his blood pressure medication after 30+ years. Focusing together on their ongoing health and well-being can do wonders for their relationship.

Final Thoughts for Men

If you're a man reading this, know you can achieve incredible results with this program. You may find that self-hypnosis comes more easily to you, so I encourage you to make it a daily habit. It's a powerful tool to enhance your focus and help you achieve your goals faster.

If you're a woman reading this, and you want to help a man in your life get healthier, don't just tell him what to do, show him. Please share this book, encourage him to join you, or simply start following the method yourself. He'll notice your success and want to get on board. If he starts to release weight faster than you, remind yourself that everyone's journey is unique. This is not a competition; always treat your experience with grace and appreciation.

Men may release weight faster than women, but that doesn't mean their journey is any less meaningful. Whether you're here for health, energy, or confidence, this program will support you in achieving and maintaining your goals for life.

You Are a Warrior — Your Journey Is Real!

ProTip: Men, use your natural focus and determination to your advantage. Stick to the plan, celebrate progress, and let your competitive edge drive you. For couples, work as a team, support and motivate each other. Remember, this journey isn't a race; it's about building a healthier, stronger future.

You Are a Warrior — Your Journey Is Real!

My Journey

Are there men in your life that you wish would pay more attention to their health? What are three ways you can help empower them to WANT to get healthier?

_____

_____

_____

_____

_____

_____

_____

_____

_____

_____

_____

_____

_____

_____

CHAPTER 29

For the Kids

"Today you are You, that is truer than true. There is no one alive who is Youer than You!" — Dr. Seuss, *Happy Birthday to You!*

"You have brains in your head. You have feet in your shoes. You can steer yourself any direction you choose." — Dr. Seuss, *Oh, the Places You'll Go!*

I struggled with writing this chapter. My intention is not to body shame, ridicule, or pass judgment on any child or parent. Having grown up being made fun of, I know the damage kids can do to each other. Not just kids, but adults, too, have a subtle way of "suggesting" that maybe you've had enough to eat or hinting that the broccoli would be a better choice than the potato. And then there's the quiet, almost whispered conversations about a child's weight that kids inevitably overhear. Let's be clear: none of this helps. But neither does the normalization or acceptance of childhood obesity as just another part of growing up.

From 2017 to March 2020, the prevalence of obesity among U.S. children and adolescents was 19.7%. This means nearly 14.7 million kids, aged 2–19 years, are now classified as obese. Thinking back to my own childhood, I was the fattest kid in my K–12 classes. Back then, I felt so alone in my struggle. But today, I'd be far from the only one. Obesity among kids aged 6–11 has more than tripled over the decades, rising from 4.2% in the 1960s to 15.3% by 2000. These numbers aren't just statistics; they're a wake-up call.

It only takes a trip to a restaurant, strip mall, amusement park, schoolyard, or any place kids gather to see the effects of our American diet. Just the other day, I was watching a football game. I couldn't believe the Frosted Flakes commercial tugging at our collective nostalgia, convincing parents to stock up on sugary cereals for breakfast. And Pop-Tarts? I remember those well, blueberry and strawberry, even before they had icing. But haven't we already seen the long-term results of the breakfasts we grew up on in the '60s, '70s, and beyond?

This isn't just about what we see; it's about what we know. I am heartbroken when I see commercials for medications and insulin devices aimed at young people. Yes, it's incredible that we have apps and tools to manage diabetes, but is that the future we want for our kids? A lifetime of managing preventable health conditions because of the habits we allowed them to form.

I understand the struggle; it's real. Between school dropoffs, soccer practices, and the daily hustle of working parents, it's easy to fall into the convenience trap. My son was definitely a product of Happy Meals, Kraft Mac & Cheese, and all the other quick, easy meals that were so popular when he was growing up.

Thankfully, he now cares about his health. He works out, trains for marathons, and watches his diet.

But I get it: convenience often feels like the only option. The truth, though, is that what's marketed as "convenient" is frequently a trap. The Frosted Flakes and Pop-Tarts of our childhood didn't do us any favors, and today's options aren't any better. Processed foods are loaded with sugar, unhealthy fats, and additives that keep kids craving more. Food companies know precisely what they're doing, banking on our nostalgia and busy schedules to keep profits high. Have you ever seen apples and oranges by the checkout counter? Fortunately, with self-checkout, we are less likely to be tempted by the candy facing us and our kids.

The good news is, we're not powerless. As parents, grandparents, aunts, uncles, and caregivers, we can rewrite the script for this generation. Small, manageable changes can make a big difference. Swap out sugary drinks for water or milk. Offer fruits or veggies instead of chips. Involve kids in the kitchen, it's excellent how much more willing they are to try new foods when they've helped prepare them.

But let's not stop with food. Movement matters, too. Kids don't need structured gym routines; they just need to move. Whether riding bikes, playing tag, or jumping on a trampoline, the goal is to get them off the couch and away from screens.

Remember when we played outside until the streetlights came on? Let's bring some of that back.

I remember building snow forts, hanging out, and walking on Ocean Parkway with my friends. Obviously, I could have done with a lot more physical activity, but I had already been emotionally damaged by being ridiculed. My wish would be for no other child to experience that shame, depression, and lack of confidence.

And here's the thing: promoting body positivity and self-acceptance is essential; every child deserves to feel loved and valued, no matter their size. But self-acceptance doesn't mean ignoring the health risks that come with obesity. Loving our kids means helping them be the healthiest versions of themselves. Sometimes, that means tough conversations and making changes as a family.

So, where do we start? Awareness is key. Pay attention to food labels; if sugar or corn syrup is one of the first ingredients, think twice. Plan meals when you can, and don't be afraid to say no to junk food.

Just like you embraced balance in your Freedom Eater 80/20 lifestyle, our kids can benefit from a similar approach. Teaching them that treats, and convenience foods can be enjoyed in moderation sets them up for a lifetime of healthy habits, without feeling deprived.

Hypnosis can be a powerful tool with kids. They do not have nearly as much judgment or baggage clouding their minds. Seek out a professional hypnotist or hypnotherapist (terminology varies by State law). It might be just the thing for a challenged eater or a kid who won't get off the couch. I have worked with teenagers on study habits with tremendous results.

By making small changes, we're not just helping our kids but setting the stage for a healthier, more vibrant future for generations. This isn't about perfection but progress, one step at a time. Together, we can rewrite the story. They are Warriors; Their Journey is Real!

> ***ProTip***: Helping kids establish healthy habits starts with minor changes. Swap sugary drinks for water, introduce fruits and veggies as snacks, and involve them in meal prep to make healthy eating fun. Encourage movement through

play, biking, tag, or running around the yard. Balance is key: treats in moderation and nutritious meals should be the norm. Hypnosis can be a powerful tool for kids. Together, we can create a future where our kids thrive. They are Warriors; Their Journey is Real!

My Journey

Are there children or teenagers in your life who you feel are over-weight and potentially headed for health concerns? What are three ways you can make a difference in their lifestyle?

_____

_____

_____

_____

_____

_____

_____

_____

_____

_____

_____

_____

_____

_____

CHAPTER 30

It's a Wrap

"There are far, far better things ahead than any we leave behind." — C.S. Lewis

---

You've made it. The end of this book and, hopefully, the beginning of a lifelong journey of self-discovery that never truly ends. If you're now at a place of comfort with your Ideal Healthy Weight, my heartfelt congratulations, I am so proud of you. Hang in there if you're still on your way to that goal.

You Are a Warrior — Your Journey Is Real!

Remember the tools you've learned, your self-hypnosis techniques, your newfound understanding of food and movement, and the chapters that resonated most with you. Go back to them when you need a boost. Let this book be your accountability partner, cheerleader, and guide when the path feels challenging.

My goal in writing this book was not just to give you the 30 to Life Program but to share my journey, which spanned over 50 years of self-doubt, self-recrimination, and the constant cycle of dieting, losing, gaining, and feeling stuck. What a crazy road trip it's been to arrive at a place where I no longer obsess about food or feel like I am always either happy with my weight or looking for the next miracle "diet." I don't start each new year thinking this is it—I'll finally get to my goal weight this time. It's taken years, but I can tell you with certainty that it's worth it.

In my work coaching women through their weight release journeys, I've seen something time and time again: a heartbreaking sense of failure. After countless diets, drugs, and even surgeries, the toll these attempts take goes far beyond physical health. Add in the hormonal upheaval of perimenopause, menopause, and post-menopause, and you've got a recipe for frustration, depression, and feeling completely out of control. It's scary, and likely contributing to an increase in female suicides.

Who is this woman who snaps at everyone? Where did this excess weight come from? Why has the scale suddenly refused to budge, no matter what I do? If you've asked yourself these questions, you're not alone. And let me assure you, it's not your fault.

But here's the good news: we can stop the madness, the endless striving to release those last ten pounds, the guilt, the deprivation, the feeling that your worth is tied to the size of your jeans or the number on the scale.

What if you instead focused on balancing your hormones and trusting your body to find its Ideal Healthy Weight? What if you learned that no food is truly off-limits (unless you're allergic), as long as you understand your physical and emotional relationship with it? What if you stopped chasing perfection and embraced progress, however small, as the incredible win that it is?

What if you could stop comparing yourself incessantly with friends, celebrities, and magazine models?

I used to look at thin women eating in restaurants and think, "Why can't that be me? She doesn't seem to have any issue with staying slim." Now, my perspective has shifted. I no longer see those women as competitors or symbols of unattainable perfection. Instead, I see women who may also struggle to see their value beyond a number on the scale. And that's where my heart lies, helping those who want to live a thinner, healthier lifestyle but feel lost on how to make that last.

You picked up this book, and I so appreciate that you did. Whether the information is meant for you or someone else you care about, I know another woman (or man) is reaching for that place of self-awareness and self-love that too often revolves around what we see in the mirror. I hope many youngsters will also learn healthier, sustainable eating that will last a lifetime.

For those using new prescription drugs to release weight, this book is a guide to what comes next. How will you maintain your weight release once the prescription ends? Will you stay on the drug indefinitely? And most importantly, have you taken the time to reflect on your relationship with food and how it affects your health, mindset, and life? These questions are critical because true, lasting change comes from understanding yourself—your triggers, habits, and emotions around food —and learning to work with your body instead of against it.

So, let's rewrite the narrative. You are so much more than a number or a size. You are worthy of love, respect, and care just as you are right now. This journey isn't about reaching perfection but finding peace with yourself and your body.

Remember, this is your journey, and every step you take matters. You're worth it, and you've got this. Be that Warrior – Honor Your Journey!

> ***ProTip*** – Water and Walking are my absolute go-tos. Once you make movement a habit and drink half your body weight in ounces of water daily, you will crave both.

I want you to experience what it's like to be a Freedom Eater. Please reach out to me at <u>Debbie@30toLife.org</u>. Remember to visit my Free Resources Page <u>https://30toLife.org</u>. For more guidance, support, and accountability, and to support other women, join our Balanced Warrior Community.

My Journey

What did you learn about your relationship to food? How has your weight affected your perception of yourself and the world? Describe what committing to your ideal healthy weight, movement, and mindset has done for your confidence.

_____

_____

_____

_____

_____

_____

_____

_____

_____

_____

_____

_____

_____

CHAPTER 31

15 Quick Tips

"Success is the sum of small efforts, repeated day in and day out." — Robert Collier

---

1. Practice "Crowding Out" Instead of Cutting Out

Fill your plate with non-starchy vegetables first, leaving less room for starchy, sugary, or fatty foods. This method makes healthier eating feel less restrictive.

2. Prep for Success

Prepare meals in advance to avoid unhealthy choices. Pack balanced lunches for work or babysitting and keep healthy snacks on hand to reduce temptation.

3. Balance Hydration

Drink half your body weight in ounces of water daily (up to 100 ounces). Start early in the day to avoid frequent bathroom trips at night.

4. Use Self-Hypnosis

At night, repeat affirmations like, "Every day, in every way, I am better and better," 10 times to program your subconscious with positive suggestions.

5. Embrace Non-Scale Victories

Focus on wins like improved energy, better sleep, clearer skin, and reduced brain fog, not just the number on the scale.

6. Avoid Trigger Foods

Identify foods you can't stop eating (e.g., chips, cashews). Avoid buying them, or portion them into single servings to control intake.

7. Read Labels Carefully

Watch for misleading terms like "All Natural." Check the ingredient list to avoid added sugars, salts, or processed additives.

8. Plan for Social Situations

Look up restaurant menus in advance or ask hosts about meal plans. Be honest about your preferences, but don't stress if options are limited.

9. Never Say Never

No food is off-limits forever. Occasionally, enjoy your favorite treats mindfully. Total restriction can lead to overindulgence.

10. Find Movement You Love

Incorporate gentle activities like walking, dancing, or yoga during the Balanced Warrior phase. Avoid high-intensity workouts to keep cortisol levels in check. Certain high-intensity exercise puts stress on the body, which can raise cortisol. While this is generally good, it is not beneficial when balancing your hormones.

11. Reward Yourself Non-Food Ways

Celebrate your progress with a manicure, new clothing, or a kitchen gadget, not with food. Focus on non-food-based rewards to reinforce positive habits.

12. Be Patient During Detox

Detox symptoms like headaches or fatigue during the Balanced Warrior 30-day balancing phase are temporary. Rest, hydrate, and stay consistent.

13. Ditch "Lose"—Use "Release"

Train your subconscious by saying you're "releasing weight" rather than "losing weight." Your subconscious won't look for what it believes is "released instead of lost."

14. Log Your Progress

Use your 30-Day Balanced Warrior Journal to track daily weight, meals, and notes on how your body responds to different foods. This will help you identify patterns and celebrate progress.

15. The Freedom Eater 80/20 Rule for Maintenance

Once balanced, aim for 80% healthy eating and 20% indulgence. Stick to veggies, water, and movement during your 80%, and enjoy treats during your 20%.

YOU ARE A WARRIOR

YOUR JOURNEY IS REAL!

My Journey

Which quick tips resonate most with you? Write about one or two that you can immediately incorporate into your daily routine.

_____

_____

_____

_____

_____

_____

_____

_____

_____

_____

_____

_____

_____

_____

_____

PART 8

RECIPES

CHAPTER 32

Recipes – Balanced Warrior 30-Day Balancing

"You don't have to cook fancy or complicated masterpieces— just good food from fresh ingredients."
—Julia Child

One of the most common questions I get asked is about recipes for the first Balanced Warrior phase and beyond, while you work toward your goal weight. I do not cook, never learned. My mom didn't cook much, and my grandmother, though she made hearty meals, focused on managing her Type I diabetes, which meant dinners were often simple and, well, bland. All the men in my life have been great cooks. As I mentioned, mother frequently reminds me that "necessity is the mother of invention."

I've tried to cook because it seems like it would be fun to be good at it. But here's the thing: I get distracted. I'll start cooking, put something on the stove, and get involved in five other things simultaneously. Let's say it's not a great recipe for success! I make an awesome pot of coffee and am always amazed by those who can create such magnificent meals.

For those who do cook and enjoy the process, these 25 recipes for your Balanced Warrior phase will guide you through the first 30 days of hormone balancing and onward to your goal. Remember, this is about living your life diet-free. You're eating real, wholesome food, and the best part? Family members can enjoy these recipes right alongside you.

We've had many couples where only one partner committed to the program, but without exception, the other partner also started releasing weight by simply eating along with the plan. The bonus? You'll save money by eating more intentionally, especially in those first 30 days.

So grab your apron—or not—and let's dive in. Whether you're an experienced chef or a reluctant cook like me, these recipes are designed to make your journey enjoyable and sustainable.

You will also find recipes for after the Balanced Warrior phase. These recipes include creative ideas for Breakfast, Lunch, Dinner, and Dessert, offering delicious and satisfying ways to maintain your progress while enjoying the journey. As you experiment, I'd love for you to share your recipes on our social media pages or email me at Debbie@30toLife.org.

Balanced Warrior
30-Day Balancing Recipes

Zucchini Noodles with Tomato Basil Sauce

Portion Size: Serves 1

Ingredients:
- 1 medium zucchini (uncooked, spiralized into noodles)
- 1 cup crushed tomatoes (no added oil or sugar)
- 2 fresh basil leaves, chopped
- 1 garlic clove, minced
- Salt and pepper to taste

Instructions:
1. Heat the crushed tomatoes and garlic in a pan over medium heat for 5 minutes.
2. Add the chopped basil, salt, and pepper. Cook for another 2 minutes.

3. Pour the sauce over the zucchini noodles. Toss gently to coat.

Tip: Use a spiralizer to create uniform zucchini noodles. If you don't have one, a vegetable peeler makes ribbons as well.

Cucumber & Dill Salad

Portion Size: Serves 1

Ingredients:
- 1 medium cucumber, thinly sliced
- 2 tablespoons lemon juice
- 1 tablespoon fresh dill, chopped
- 1/4 teaspoon salt

Instructions:

1. Toss the cucumber slices with lemon juice, dill, and salt in a bowl.

2. Let it chill in the fridge for 10 minutes before serving.

Tip: Add a few slices of radish or celery for an extra crunch.

Roasted Cauliflower "Steaks"

Portion Size: Serves 1

Ingredients:
- 1 large cauliflower, cut into thick slices (like steaks)
- 1 teaspoon paprika
- 1 teaspoon garlic powder
- 1 teaspoon onion powder

- Salt to taste

Instructions:

1. Preheat your oven to 400°F (200°C).

2. Sprinkle paprika, garlic powder, onion powder, and salt over the cauliflower slices.

3. Roast on a baking sheet lined with parchment paper for 2025 minutes or until tender and golden.

Tip: Cauliflower "steaks" make a hearty and satisfying meat substitute for plant-based meals.

Spaghetti Squash Bowl with Veggies

Portion Size: Serves 1

Ingredients:

- 1/2 spaghetti squash (cooked and scraped into strands)
- 1 cup steamed broccoli
- 1/2 cup diced cherry tomatoes
- 1 teaspoon garlic powder
- Salt and pepper to taste

Instructions:

1. Toss the spaghetti squash strands with garlic powder, salt, and pepper.

2. Top with steamed broccoli and diced tomatoes.

Tip: Bake the spaghetti squash at 375°F (190°C) for 40 minutes for perfectly tender strands.

Lemon-Ginger Steamed Asparagus

Portion Size: Serves 1

Ingredients:
- 1 cup fresh asparagus spears
- 1 teaspoon grated ginger
- 1 tablespoon lemon juice

Instructions:
1. Steam the asparagus for 5-7 minutes until tender.
2. Toss with grated ginger and lemon juice before serving.

Tip: Add a pinch of sea salt to enhance the natural flavors.

Tomato & Herb Gazpacho

Portion Size: Serves 1

Ingredients:
- 2 medium tomatoes, chopped
- 1/2 cucumber, chopped
- 1/4 red bell pepper, chopped
- 1 teaspoon fresh parsley
- 1 teaspoon fresh cilantro
- 1 tablespoon lime juice

Instructions:

1. Blend all ingredients in a blender until smooth.

2. Chill for 30 minutes before serving.

Tip: Garnish with a cucumber slice or fresh parsley for an elegant presentation.

Simple Celery Sticks with Salsa

Portion Size: Serves 1

Ingredients:

- 4 celery sticks, cut into 3-inch pieces
- 1/4 cup fresh salsa (no oil or sugar added)

Instructions:

1. Serve the celery sticks with salsa for dipping.

Tip: Use a chunky salsa for more texture and flavor. Remember to check for added sugar on the label.

Steamed Spinach & Lemon

Portion Size: Serves 1

Ingredients:

- 2 cups fresh spinach leaves
- 1 tablespoon lemon juice
- 1 garlic clove, minced

Instructions:

1. Steam the spinach for 3-5 minutes, just until wilted.

2. Toss with lemon juice and minced garlic before serving.

Tip: Don't over-steam the spinach; it should still be vibrant green. If you need more greens to crowd out something else, have more than 2 cups. Fill your plate with greens.

Cauliflower Mash with Garlic

Portion Size: Serves 1

Ingredients:

- 1 cup steamed cauliflower florets
- 1 garlic clove, roasted
- Salt to taste

Instructions:

1. Blend the steamed cauliflower and roasted garlic in a blender or food processor until smooth.

2. Add salt to taste and serve warm.

Tip: Add a dash of nutmeg for a unique flavor twist.

Rainbow Veggie Lettuce Wraps

Portion Size: Serves 1

Ingredients:

- 2 large romaine lettuce leaves

- 1/4 cup shredded carrots

- 1/4 cup diced red bell pepper

- 1/4 cup cucumber, julienned

- 1 teaspoon lime juice

Instructions:

1. Layer the veggies on the lettuce leaves.

2. Drizzle with lime juice and roll up tightly to eat like a wrap.

Tip: Add fresh cilantro for an extra burst of flavor.

Grilled Portobello Mushroom "Steak"

Portion Size: Serves 1

Ingredients:

- 1 large Portobello mushroom cap

- 1 teaspoon garlic powder

- 1 teaspoon smoked paprika

- Salt to taste

Instructions:

1. Preheat a grill pan or outdoor grill.

2. Sprinkle the mushroom cap with garlic powder, smoked paprika, and salt.

3. Grill for 5-7 minutes on each side, or until tender.

Tip: Portobello mushrooms have a meaty texture that makes them a satisfying main dish.

Carrot & Ginger Soup

Portion Size: Serves 1

Ingredients:
- 1 medium carrot, peeled and chopped
- 1 cup vegetable broth (low sodium)
- 1 teaspoon grated ginger
- Salt to taste

Instructions:
1. Boil the chopped carrot in vegetable broth until soft.
2. Blend the soup with the grated ginger until smooth.
3. Add salt to taste and serve warm.

Tip: Garnish with a sprinkle of fresh parsley or a dollop of plain Greek yogurt—skip the yogurt in the first 30 days.

Steamed Green Beans with Lemon Zest

Portion Size: Serves 1

Ingredients:
- 1 cup green beans, trimmed
- 1 teaspoon lemon zest
- Salt to taste

Instructions:
1. Steam the green beans for 7-10 minutes or until tender crisp.

2. Sprinkle with lemon zest and salt before serving.

Tip: Serve alongside a lean protein for a balanced meal.

Cabbage Stir-Fry

Portion Size: Serves 1

Ingredients:
- 1 cup shredded cabbage
- 1 garlic clove, minced
- 1 tablespoon low-sodium vegetable broth
- Salt to taste

Instructions:
1. Heat a nonstick pan and add the vegetable broth and garlic.
2. Toss in the shredded cabbage and stir-fry for 5-7 minutes.
3. Add salt to taste and serve warm.

Tip: Add a splash of apple cider vinegar for a tangy kick. I choose organic broth. If you can, do that.

Roasted Brussels Sprouts with Apple Cider Vinegar

Portion Size: Serves 1

Ingredients:
- 1 cup Brussels sprouts, halved
- 1 tablespoon apple cider vinegar

- Salt to taste

Instructions:

1. Preheat the oven to 400°F (200°C).

2. Toss the halved Brussels sprouts with apple cider vinegar and salt.

3. Roast on a parchment-lined baking sheet for 20 minutes, flipping halfway.

Tip: For extra flavor, sprinkle freshly cracked pepper before serving. You can always add a drop of plain liquid Stevia to sweeten just a bit.

Chilled Cucumber & Lime Salad

Portion Size: Serves 1

Ingredients:

- 1 medium cucumber, thinly sliced

- 1 tablespoon lime juice

- 1 teaspoon chopped fresh cilantro

- Salt to taste

Instructions:

1. Toss the cucumber slices with lime juice, cilantro, and salt in a bowl.

2. Chill in the refrigerator for 10 minutes before serving.

Tip: This is a quick and refreshing side dish for summer meals. Fresh lime only.

Roasted Zucchini with Garlic

Portion Size: Serves 1

Ingredients:
- 1 medium zucchini, sliced into rounds
- 1 garlic clove, minced
- 1 teaspoon dried oregano
- Salt and pepper to taste

Instructions:
1. Preheat the oven to 375°F (190°C).
2. Arrange zucchini slices on a baking sheet lined with parchment paper.
3. Sprinkle with minced garlic, oregano, salt, and pepper.
4. Roast for 15-20 minutes or until tender.

Tip: Zucchini is a low-calorie vegetable that absorbs flavors beautifully. It's also a great one in an air fryer.

Sautéed Spinach with Mushrooms

Portion Size: Serves 1

Ingredients:
- 2 cups fresh spinach leaves
- 1/2 cup sliced mushrooms
- 1 garlic clove, minced

- 1 tablespoon low-sodium vegetable broth
- Salt and pepper to taste

Instructions:

1. Heat the vegetable broth in a nonstick pan over medium heat.
2. Add the garlic and mushrooms, cooking for 3-4 minutes.
3. Toss in the spinach and cook until just wilted. Season with salt and pepper.

Tip: This dish pairs well with grilled chicken or tofu.

Lemon-Baked Sole

Portion Size: Serves 1

Ingredients:

- 1 sole fillet
- 1 tablespoon lemon juice
- 1 teaspoon dried dill
- Salt and pepper to taste

Instructions:

1. Preheat the oven to 375°F (190°C).
2. Place the sole fillet on a parchment-lined baking sheet.
3. Drizzle with lemon juice and sprinkle with dill, salt, and pepper.
4. Bake for 10-12 minutes or until the fish flakes easily with a fork.

Tip: Serve with steamed broccoli or asparagus for a complete meal.

Sweet Pepper & Herb Soup

Portion Size: Serves 1

Ingredients:
- 1 red bell pepper, roasted and peeled
- 1 cup vegetable broth (low sodium). Choose organic, if possible.
- 1 garlic clove, minced
- 1 teaspoon fresh thyme leaves
- Salt and pepper to taste

Instructions:
1. Blend the roasted red bell pepper with the vegetable broth, garlic, and thyme until smooth.
2. Heat the soup in a pot over medium heat, seasoning with salt and pepper.
3. Serve warm with a garnish of fresh thyme.

Tip: Roasting the bell pepper enhances its natural sweetness, making this soup irresistibly flavorful.

Herb-Crusted Tilapia

Portion Size: Serves 1

Ingredients:
- 1 tilapia fillet
- 1 teaspoon dried oregano

- 1 teaspoon garlic powder

- Zest of 1 lemon

- Salt and pepper to taste

Instructions:
1. Preheat the oven to 375°F (190°C).

2. Mix oregano, garlic powder, and lemon zest in a small bowl.

3. Sprinkle the mixture evenly over the tilapia fillet and season with salt and pepper.

4. Place the fillet on a parchment-lined baking sheet and bake for 10-12 minutes.

Tip: Serve with steamed green beans for a complete meal. I have not been able to find wild-caught tilapia, but don't stress if you need to use farm-raised.

Cucumber & Mint Salad

Portion Size: Serves 1

Ingredients:
- 1 medium cucumber, thinly sliced

- 1 tablespoon fresh mint leaves, chopped

- 1 tablespoon lime juice

- Pinch of salt

Instructions:
1. Toss cucumber slices with chopped mint, lime juice, and a pinch of salt.

2. Chill in the refrigerator for 10 minutes before serving.

Tip: This refreshing salad pairs well with grilled fish or chicken.

Steamed Broccoli with Garlic

Portion Size: Serves 1

Ingredients:
- 1 cup broccoli florets
- 1 garlic clove, minced
- 1 tablespoon low-sodium vegetable broth
- Salt to taste

Instructions:
1. Steam the broccoli for 5-7 minutes until tender but crisp.
2. In a small pan, heat the vegetable broth and sauté the garlic for 1 minute.
3. Drizzle the garlic sauce over the broccoli before serving.

Tip: Add a squeeze of lemon for extra brightness.

Zesty Carrot Slaw

Portion Size: Serves 1

Ingredients:
- 1 medium carrot, shredded
- 1 teaspoon lime juice

- 1 teaspoon fresh cilantro, chopped
- Salt to taste

Instructions:
1. Toss the shredded carrot with lime juice, cilantro, and a pinch of salt.
2. Serve immediately, or let it chill in the fridge for added flavor.

Tip: This slaw is a crunchy topping for lettuce wraps or grilled fish.

Roasted Cherry Tomatoes with Thyme

Portion Size: Serves 1

Ingredients:
- 1 cup cherry tomatoes
- 1 teaspoon fresh thyme leaves
- Salt and pepper to taste

Instructions:
1. Preheat the oven to 400°F (200°C).
2. Place cherry tomatoes on a parchment-lined baking sheet.
3. Sprinkle with thyme, salt, and pepper.
4. Roast 15-20 minutes or until the tomatoes are soft and slightly caramelized.

Tip: Use these roasted tomatoes as a topping for zucchini noodles or as a side dish.

CHAPTER 33

Recipes – Harmony Heroine – Reintroducing Foods

By now, your body has had the opportunity to reset and recalibrate, and you've likely started noticing positive changes in your energy level, mindset, and overall well-being. After the balancing, the Harmony Heroine phase is all about reintroducing a variety of wholesome, nutrient-dense foods while continuing to work toward your Ideal Healthy Weight.

This phase allows for more flexibility, incorporating healthy fats, starchy vegetables, and grains into your meals. The goal remains the same: enjoying satisfying food that nourishes your body and supports your journey. These recipes are designed to fit seamlessly into your life, whether you're dining solo or feeding the whole family. Please check the recipe to be sure you have already reintroduced all the foods. You can certainly reintroduce a particular food by making one of the recipes; however, be sure all the other ingredients have already been reintroduced.

To simplify, I've divided the recipes into categories— Breakfast, Lunch, Dinner, and Dessert. Start your day with energizing breakfasts, fuel up with balanced lunches, savor satisfying dinners, and treat yourself to guilt-free desserts. Let these recipes inspire your culinary creativity and help you continue building a sustainable, healthy lifestyle.

Let's dive into these delicious recipes that celebrate the joy of eating well!

NOTE: Each recipe is one serving.

BREAKFASTS

Avocado Toast with Cherry Tomatoes

Ingredients
- 1 slice whole-grain bread, toasted
- 1/2 ripe avocado, mashed
- 4 cherry tomatoes, halved
- 1 teaspoon olive oil
- Salt and pepper to taste

Instructions
1. Spread mashed avocado over the toasted bread.
2. Top with halved cherry tomatoes and drizzle with olive oil.
3. Sprinkle with salt and pepper.

Helpful Tip: Add a sprinkle of chili flakes for a spicy twist!

Anecdote: Avocado toast became a worldwide breakfast sensation after Instagram blew up with creative toast photos. It's a millennial breakfast staple for good reason!

Greek Yogurt Parfait with Berries

Ingredients
- 1 cup plain Greek yogurt
- 1/4 cup fresh blueberries
- 1/4 cup fresh strawberries, sliced
- 2 tablespoons granola (low sugar)
- 1 teaspoon honey (optional)

Instructions
1. Layer yogurt, berries, and granola in a glass or bowl.
2. Drizzle with honey if desired.

Helpful Tip: Swap granola with crushed nuts for a lower-sugar alternative.

Anecdote: Did you know Greek yogurt has twice the protein of regular yogurt? It's a great way to stay full all morning. There are several dairy-free yogurts. Please be mindful of the added sugar in them (and in all yogurts).

Sweet Potato & Avocado Breakfast Bowl

Ingredients

- 1/2 roasted sweet potato, cubed
- 1/2 avocado, diced
- 1 soft-boiled egg
- 1 teaspoon olive oil
- Salt and pepper to taste

Instructions

1. Layer roasted sweet potato and avocado in a bowl.
2. Top with a soft-boiled egg and drizzle with olive oil.
3. Season with salt and pepper.

Helpful Tip: Roast sweet potatoes in bulk to save time during the week.

Anecdote: Sweet potatoes are rich in beta-carotene, which gives them their vibrant orange color and boosts your skin health!

Spinach & Feta Omelet

Ingredients

- 2 large eggs
- 1/4 cup fresh spinach, chopped
- 2 tablespoons crumbled feta cheese
- 1 teaspoon olive oil

- Salt and pepper to taste

Instructions

1. Beat the eggs and season with salt and pepper.

2. Heat olive oil in a nonstick pan and sauté spinach until wilted.

3. Add eggs to the pan, sprinkle with feta, and cook until set.

Helpful Tip: Use frozen spinach if fresh isn't available—just thaw and drain before adding.

Anecdote: Feta cheese has existed for over 8,000 years and is still traditionally made in Greece.

Banana Oat Pancakes

Ingredients

- 1 ripe banana

- 1/2 cup rolled oats

- 1 large egg

- 1/4 teaspoon cinnamon

- 1 teaspoon olive oil

Instructions

1. Blend the banana, oats, egg, and cinnamon until smooth.

2. Heat olive oil in a nonstick pan and pour batter into small pancake rounds.

3. Cook for 2-3 minutes on each side until golden.

Helpful Tip: Add fresh fruit or a dollop of Greek yogurt on top for extra flavor.

Anecdote: This recipe is a lifesaver for using up overripe bananas, no waste, all taste!

LUNCHES

Quinoa & Avocado Salad Bowl

Ingredients
- 1/2 cup cooked quinoa
- 1/2 avocado, sliced
- 1/2 cup cherry tomatoes, halved
- 1/4 cup cucumber, diced
- 1 tablespoon olive oil
- 1 tablespoon lemon juice
- Salt and pepper to taste

Instructions
1. Layer quinoa, avocado, cherry tomatoes, and cucumber in a bowl.
2. Drizzle with olive oil and lemon juice. Season with salt and pepper.

Helpful Tip: Prep a batch of quinoa at the start of the week for a quick lunch assembly.

Anecdote: Quinoa, a staple of ancient Inca warriors, is called the "mother of all grains" because it's a complete protein.

Chickpea & Spinach Wrap

Ingredients
- 1 whole-grain tortilla
- 1/2 cup cooked chickpeas
- 1/4 cup fresh spinach leaves
- 1 tablespoon hummus
- 1 teaspoon olive oil

Instructions
1. Spread hummus on the tortilla.
2. Add chickpeas, spinach, and a drizzle of olive oil. Wrap it tightly.

Helpful Tip: Warm the tortilla slightly for easier rolling.

Anecdote: Chickpeas are the base for hummus, a dip so ancient it dates to 13th-century Egypt!

Lentil & Vegetable Soup

Ingredients
- 1/2 cup cooked lentils
- 1 cup vegetable broth
- 1/4 cup diced carrots

- 1/4 cup diced celery
- 1 teaspoon olive oil
- Salt and pepper to taste

Instructions

1. Heat olive oil in a pot and sauté carrots and celery for 5 minutes.

2. Add lentils and vegetable broth. Simmer for 10 minutes.

3. Season with salt and pepper and serve warm.

Helpful Tip: Freeze small portions of lentils for quick soups like this.

Anecdote: Lentils have been a dietary staple for over 9,000 years.

They're small but mighty!

Mediterranean Veggie Bowl

Ingredients

- 1/2 cup cooked farro
- 1/4 cup diced cucumbers
- 1/4 cup diced red bell pepper
- 1 tablespoon olive oil
- 1 tablespoon lemon juice
- 2 tablespoons crumbled feta cheese

Instructions

1. Combine farro, cucumbers, and red bell pepper in a bowl.

2. Drizzle with olive oil and lemon juice, and sprinkle feta cheese on top.

Helpful Tip: Substitute farro with brown rice or barley if needed. Faro is an ancient whole grain-like barley with a nutty flavor, a chewy texture, and a subtle sweetness, often used in soups, salads, and grain bowls. I didn't know what farro was until I ordered a veggie bowl with it in a restaurant. Change up your grains and experiment.

Anecdote: Farro has been cultivated for over 10,000 years and was a favorite of Roman soldiers.

Smashed Avocado & Chickpea Salad Sandwich

Ingredients
- 2 slices whole-grain bread
- 1/2 avocado
- 1/4 cup cooked chickpeas, mashed
- 1 teaspoon lemon juice
- Salt and pepper to taste

Instructions
1. Mash avocado and chickpeas together in a bowl.
2. Add lemon juice, salt, and pepper, then spread on bread slices.

Helpful Tip: Toast the bread for extra crunch and flavor.

Anecdote: Avocado and chickpeas are a dream team, creamy, filling, and packed with nutrients.

DINNERS

Lemon Herb Grilled Chicken with Quinoa

Ingredients

- 1 chicken breast, grilled
- 1/2 cup cooked quinoa
- 1 tablespoon olive oil
- 1 tablespoon lemon juice
- 1/2 teaspoon dried thyme
- Salt and pepper to taste

Instructions

1. Marinate the chicken breast with olive oil, lemon juice, thyme, salt, and pepper.
2. Grill the chicken for 6-8 minutes per side or until fully cooked.
3. Serve over a bed of quinoa.

Helpful Tip: Pounding the chicken breast to an even thickness ensures it cooks evenly.

Anecdote: Lemon and thyme are a match made in culinary heaven, and they make chicken anything but boring!

Sweet Potato & Black Bean Chili

Ingredients

- 1/2 cup diced sweet potato
- 1/2 cup cooked black beans
- 1 cup diced tomatoes (canned or fresh)
- 1 teaspoon chili powder
- 1 teaspoon smoked paprika
- Salt to taste

Instructions

1. Heat a pot and sauté sweet potato with a bit of water for 5 minutes.
2. Add tomatoes, black beans, chili powder, paprika, and salt.

Simmer for 10 minutes.

Helpful Tip: Add a squeeze of lime for a zesty finish.

Anecdote: Black beans are sometimes called "turtle beans" because of their shiny, dark appearance!

Salmon with Avocado Salsa

Ingredients

- 1 salmon fillet – look for wild caught if your budget permits
- 1/2 avocado, diced
- 1 tablespoon lime juice 1 tablespoon olive oil
- Salt and pepper to taste

Instructions

1. Season the salmon with olive oil, salt, and pepper. Bake at 375°F (190°C) for 12-15 minutes.

2. Combine diced avocado with lime juice to make a salsa.

3. Top the salmon with avocado salsa before serving.

Helpful Tip: If you're short on time, cook the salmon in a pan instead of the oven.

Anecdote: Salmon is rich in omega-3 fatty acids, which are essential for brain health—food for thought, literally!

Veggie Stir-Fry with Brown Rice

Ingredients

- 1/2 cup cooked brown rice 1/2 cup broccoli florets

- 1/4 cup sliced bell peppers

- 1/4 cup snap peas

- 1 teaspoon olive oil

- 1 teaspoon soy sauce (low sodium)

Instructions

1. Heat olive oil in a nonstick pan and sauté broccoli, bell peppers, and snap peas for 5 minutes.

2. Add soy sauce and toss to coat. Serve over brown rice.

Helpful Tip: Prep your veggies ahead of time to make this a quick weeknight meal.

Anecdote: Snap peas are nature's crunchy snack, they even "snap" when you break them in half!

Baked Cod with Lemon & Dill

Ingredients

- 1 cod fillet
- 1 tablespoon olive oil
- 1 tablespoon lemon juice
- 1 teaspoon dried dill
- Salt and pepper to taste

Instructions

1. Drizzle the cod fillet with olive oil and lemon juice.
2. Sprinkle with dill, salt, and pepper.
3. Bake at 375°F (190°C) for 10-12 minutes or until flaky.

Helpful Tip: For a balanced plate, serve with steamed asparagus or green beans.

Anecdote: Cod has been a culinary favorite for centuries and was even a staple food during Viking expeditions!

Quinoa Stuffed Bell Peppers

Ingredients

- 1 large bell pepper, halved and de-seeded
- 1/2 cup cooked quinoa
- 1/4 cup diced tomatoes
- 1/4 cup black beans

- 1 teaspoon chili powder

Instructions

1. Mix quinoa, tomatoes, black beans, and chili powder in a bowl.

2. Stuff the mixture into the bell pepper halves.

3. Bake at 375°F (190°C) for 20 minutes.

Helpful Tip: Use different-colored peppers for a more vibrant dish. Green peppers do not work for me, but I always have orange, red, and yellow, which are great in salads, too.

Anecdote: Bell peppers are technically fruits, not vegetables, just like tomatoes!

Roasted Veggie & Chickpea Bowl

Ingredients

- 1/2 cup roasted sweet potato cubes

- 1/2 cup roasted broccoli

- 1/2 cup cooked chickpeas

- 1 tablespoon olive oil

- 1 teaspoon smoked paprika

Instructions

1. Toss the sweet potato, broccoli, and chickpeas with olive oil and smoked paprika.

2. Roast at 400°F (200°C) for 20-25 minutes, tossing halfway through.

Helpful Tip: Add a dollop of hummus for extra creaminess.

Anecdote: Roasted veggies taste so good you'll forget they're healthy!

Turkey & Zucchini Meatballs

Ingredients

- 1/4-pound ground turkey
- 1/4 cup grated zucchini
- 1 garlic clove, minced
- 1 tablespoon parsley, chopped
- Salt and pepper to taste

Instructions

1. Mix all ingredients in a bowl and form into small meatballs.
2. Bake at 375°F (190°C) for 15-20 minutes, flipping halfway through.

Helpful Tip: Serve with a side of quinoa or spaghetti squash.

Anecdote: Zucchini moistens these meatballs and adds a sneaky serving of veggies!

Pasta Primavera with Whole-Wheat Pasta

Ingredients

- 1/2 cup cooked whole-wheat pasta
- 1/4 cup broccoli florets
- 1/4 cup sliced carrots

- 1/4 cup cherry tomatoes, halved
- 1 teaspoon olive oil
- 1 garlic clove, minced

Instructions

1. Heat olive oil in a pan and sauté garlic and veggies for 5 minutes.

2. Toss with cooked pasta and serve warm.

Helpful Tip: Add a sprinkle of Parmesan for extra flavor.

Anecdote: "Primavera" means "spring" in Italian, this dish is as colorful as a spring garden!

Shrimp Stir-Fry with Snap Peas

Ingredients

- 1/2 cup shrimp, peeled and deveined
- 1/2 cup snap peas
- 1 tablespoon olive oil
- 1 teaspoon soy sauce (low sodium)
- 1/2 teaspoon grated ginger

Instructions

1. Heat olive oil in a nonstick pan and sauté shrimp and snap peas for 5 minutes.

2. Add soy sauce and grated ginger. Toss to coat.

Helpful Tip: Fresh ginger freezes well—just grate it straight from the freezer!

Anecdote: Snap peas and shrimp make a perfect combo—both cook super-fast and stay crisp.

SALADS

Spinach & Strawberry Salad with Balsamic Glaze

Ingredients
- 2 cups fresh spinach leaves
- 1/2 cup fresh strawberries, sliced
- 2 tablespoons sliced almonds
- 1 tablespoon balsamic glaze

Instructions
1. Toss spinach, strawberries, and almonds in a bowl.
2. Drizzle with balsamic glaze before serving.

Helpful Tip: Toast the almonds for a nuttier flavor.

Anecdote: Strawberries and balsamic vinegar are a surprisingly perfect match, an Italian classic that works as a salad or dessert!

Mediterranean Chickpea Salad

Ingredients
- 1/2 cup cooked chickpeas
- 1/4 cup cherry tomatoes, halved
- 1/4 cup cucumber, diced

- 1 tablespoon red onion, finely chopped
- 1 tablespoon olive oil
- 1 tablespoon lemon juice
- 1 tablespoon crumbled feta cheese

Instructions

1. Combine chickpeas, tomatoes, cucumber, and red onion in a bowl.

2. Drizzle with olive oil and lemon juice, then sprinkle with feta.

Helpful Tip: This salad tastes even better if it sits for 30 minutes to let the flavors meld.

Anecdote: Chickpeas are often called "garbanzo beans," depending on where you are in the world, same legume, different names!

Kale Salad with Avocado & Sunflower Seeds

Ingredients

- 2 cups chopped kale
- 1/2 avocado, mashed
- 1 tablespoon lemon juice
- 1 tablespoon sunflower seeds
- Salt and pepper to taste

Instructions

1. Massage the kale with the mashed avocado and lemon juice until softened.

2. Top with sunflower seeds and season with salt and pepper.

Helpful Tip: Massaging kale breaks down its tough fibers, making it tender and easier to digest.

Anecdote: Kale was once just a garnish for restaurant plates, now it's a bona fide superfood star! One thing I have learned about eating kale is to have dental floss handy!

Sweet Potato & Spinach Salad

Ingredients
- 1/2 cup roasted sweet potato cubes
- 2 cups fresh spinach leaves
- 2 tablespoons dried cranberries – watch for added sugar
- 1 tablespoon olive oil
- 1 tablespoon apple cider vinegar

Instructions
1. Toss spinach, roasted sweet potato, and dried cranberries in a bowl.
2. Drizzle with olive oil and apple cider vinegar before serving.

Helpful Tip: Make extra roasted sweet potatoes for other weekly meals.

Anecdote: Dried cranberries add a sweetness that balances the earthy spinach and creamy sweet potato.

Quinoa & Roasted Veggie Salad

Ingredients

- 1/2 cup cooked quinoa
- 1/4 cup roasted zucchini
- 1/4 cup roasted bell peppers
- 1 tablespoon olive oil
- 1 tablespoon balsamic vinegar

Instructions

1. Combine quinoa, roasted zucchini, and roasted bell peppers in a bowl.
2. Drizzle with olive oil and balsamic vinegar. Toss to coat.

Helpful Tip: Roast veggies in bulk and store them in the fridge for quick meals.

Anecdote: Quinoa's versatility makes it a powerhouse for salads, bowls, and desserts!

DESSERTS – These are 20% recipes and best for after you reach your IHW (Ideal Healthy Weight)

Dark Chocolate-Dipped Strawberries

Ingredients

- 5 fresh strawberries
- 1/4 cup dark chocolate chips (70% cocoa or higher)

Instructions

1. Melt the dark chocolate chips in the microwave or a double boiler.

2. Dip the strawberries halfway into the melted chocolate.

3. Place them on parchment paper and let them set in the fridge for 10 minutes.

Helpful Tip: Add a sprinkle of sea salt or crushed nuts before the chocolate sets for extra flavor.

Anecdote: Strawberries were once a luxury fruit in France; farmers would bring them fresh to the royal court!

Baked Cinnamon Apples

Ingredients

- 1 medium apple, cored and sliced

- 1/2 teaspoon ground cinnamon

- 1 teaspoon maple syrup – if you substitute flavored liquid Stevia, I love the caramel here, you can have this during your balancing phase.

Instructions

1. Preheat your oven to 375°F (190°C).

2. Toss apple slices with cinnamon and maple syrup. You can use a maple liquid Stevia.

3. Bake for 15-20 minutes until soft and caramelized.

Helpful Tip: Serve warm with a dollop of Greek yogurt for a creamy contrast.

Anecdote: Baked apples are the perfect guilt-free dessert, bringing the warmth of a traditional apple pie without the crust!

Chia Pudding with Almond Milk

Ingredients
- 2 tablespoons chia seeds
- 1/2 cup unsweetened almond milk
- 1 teaspoon honey or maple syrup
- 1/4 cup fresh berries for topping

Instructions
1. Combine chia seeds, almond milk, and sweetener in a jar or bowl. Stir well.
2. Refrigerate for at least 2 hours or overnight.
3. Top with fresh berries before serving.

Helpful Tip: Stir the pudding after 15 minutes in the fridge to avoid clumps.

Anecdote: Chia seeds were a staple food for Aztec warriors— small but mighty in nutrients!

Coconut Banana Nice Cream

Ingredients
- 1 frozen banana, sliced
- 2 tablespoons coconut milk

Instructions

1. Blend the frozen banana and coconut milk until smooth and creamy.

2. Serve immediately as a soft-serve or freeze for 1-2 hours for a firmer texture.

Helpful Tip: Add a pinch of cinnamon or a splash of vanilla extract for extra flavor. Or vanilla liquid Stevia.

Anecdote: This "nice cream" proves that healthy desserts can be just as indulgent as their unhealthy counterparts!

Almond Butter Stuffed Dates

Ingredients

- 3 Medjool dates, pitted
- 1 tablespoon almond butter

Instructions

1. Slice the dates open lengthwise and remove the pits.

2. Fill each date with a small dollop of almond butter.

Helpful Tip: Sprinkle with shredded coconut or chopped nuts for added texture.

Anecdote: Dates are nature's candy, cultivated for over 6,000 years in the Middle East! See if you can get them organic.

Thank you for taking this journey with me.

Whether you're just starting, midway through, or already celebrating your wins, please know how proud I am of you for showing up for yourself. Deciding to reset your body, reframe your mindset, and reclaim your health is a powerful act of self-love, and I'm honored to be part of your story.

This book was created to support real people with real lives, just like you. But the journey doesn't end here. I've compiled a collection of helpful tools to keep you moving forward with ease, joy, and confidence.

Visit the FREE RESOURCES page on my website to access:

- Free downloads and printable tools
- Articles and blog posts on wellness, mindset, and hormone balance
- Details about Membership to the Balanced Warrior

Community

Details about my Private Coaching VIP Program and more ways to stay supported long after the last page. Head to https://30toLife.org (It's a page just for readers like you!)

Your next step is yours, but you never have to walk it alone.

Keep going. Keep growing.

YOU ARE A WARRIOR

YOUR JOURNEY IS REAL!

I would love to hear from you.

With gratitude,

Debbie

Debbie@30toLife.org

About the Author

Debbie Harris knows firsthand how exhausting the weight loss roller coaster can be, especially for women over 40 experiencing perimenopause or menopause, juggling hormones, careers, families, and self-care that somehow always ends up last on the list. After trying nearly every diet out there for over fifty years, and her weight going up and down, Debbie finally cracked the code on how to release weight, balance hormones, and feel confident again.

An Integrative Nutrition Health Coach, hypnotist, and the creator of the 30 to Life Solution, Debbie has helped thousands of women ditch the dieting mentality and step into lasting freedom with food. Her approach combines science, soul, and strategy, empowering women to work with their minds and bodies, not fight against them.

She's not here to sell magic pills or shame you into submission. Instead, Debbie offers real-life tools, humor, and hope to help women reclaim their energy, confidence, and joy. Her message is simple: you're not broken, you're not lazy, and it's not too late. There's a better way, and it starts with balance.

Debbie lives in Deep River, Connecticut, with her husband David, dog and two cats. She spends her time walking while listening to detective stories, traveling, writing, and laughing with clients who quickly become part of her movement to stop the dieting madness. Dieting Sucks for Women Over 40 is the book she wishes she'd had years ago, and now she's passing it on to you.

If you're struggling with your weight and want to work with someone you can trust, reach out to Debbie at https://30toLife.org.

The Book Ends Here, But Your Journey Doesn't

Thank you for making yourself a priority. I so appreciate you reading "Dieting Sucks" and making a commitment to your own health and well-being.

You Are a Warrior – Your Journey Is Real

If you felt something click, if my words resonated with you, then you already know:

This isn't just about weight. It's about freedom, clarity, energy, confidence... and yes, maybe a smaller pair of pants.

So let's keep the spark alive.

Join the Balanced Warrior Community

It's where the real-life magic happens.

Inside, you'll find the tools, the support, and the momentum to keep going, without perfection, shame, or starvation. I believe that when women lift other women, our magic is limitless.

What's Inside:

- Private group support
- Weekly prompts and resources
- Live sessions with me and other Warriors
- Real talk, real tools, real community

Scan to Join the Balanced Warrior Community Now or go to https://30toLife.org.

Use Discount Code: **WARRIOR** at checkout

Your first month is just $19 (normally $39) — because you have the book, and you are a Balanced Warrior.

With deepest gratitude, I send you my appreciation for all that you are, and all that you bring to the world. You are a gift, and no one else is YOU!

Debbie

READER BONUS!

Dear Reader,

As a thank you for your support, I would like to offer you a special reader bonus. If you've ever been on a diet and haven't been able to sustain it, this download is perfect for you.

Go to https://30toLife.org or click the QR code below and download the 30-Day Balanced Warrior Journal today.

Throughout this book, I will refer to the 30-Day Balanced Warrior Journal. Note that this is NOT a diet regimen. This is a lifestyle change. If you follow this book and commit to becoming healthy, you will. The journal is one of the many tools available to you.

Are you ready to live the life you truly want to live? Are you ready to leave that fat behind once and for all and step into your warrior phase of life? Let's do it together.

READER BONUS!

www.ingramcontent.com/pod-product-compliance
Lightning Source LLC
Chambersburg PA
CBHW070057030426
42335CB00016B/1928